the cancer diet cookbook

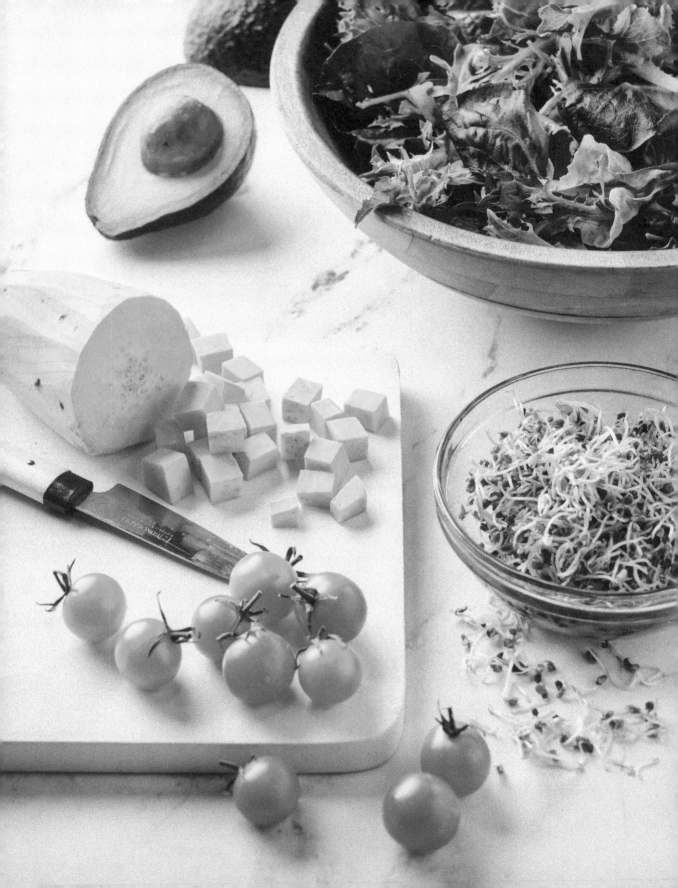

# the cancer diet cookbook

## Comforting Recipes for Treatment and Recovery

### Dionne Detraz, RDN

PHOTOGRAPHY BY THOMAS J. STORY

ROCKRIDGE
PRESS

For general information on our other products and services or to obtain technical support, please contact our Customer Care Department within the United States at (866) 744-2665, or outside the United States at (510) 253-0500.

Rockridge Press publishes its books in a variety of electronic and print formats. Some content that appears in print may not be available in electronic books, and vice versa.

Interior and Cover Designer: Angie Chiu
Art Producer: Karen Williams
Editor: Greg Morabito
Production Manager: Michael Kay
Production Editor: Sigi Nacson

Photography © 2020 Thomas J. Story
Food styling by Alexa Hyman
Cover photo: Coconut Curry Soup with Shrimp (page 106)

ISBN: Print 978-1-64739-254-3
Ebook 978-1-64739-255-0
R0

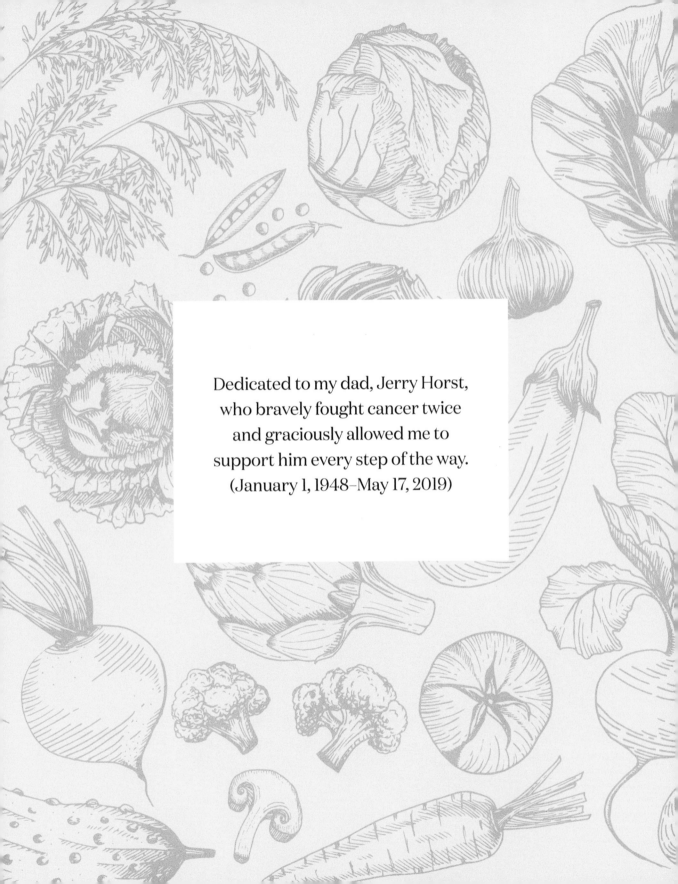

Dedicated to my dad, Jerry Horst,
who bravely fought cancer twice
and graciously allowed me to
support him every step of the way.
(January 1, 1948–May 17, 2019)

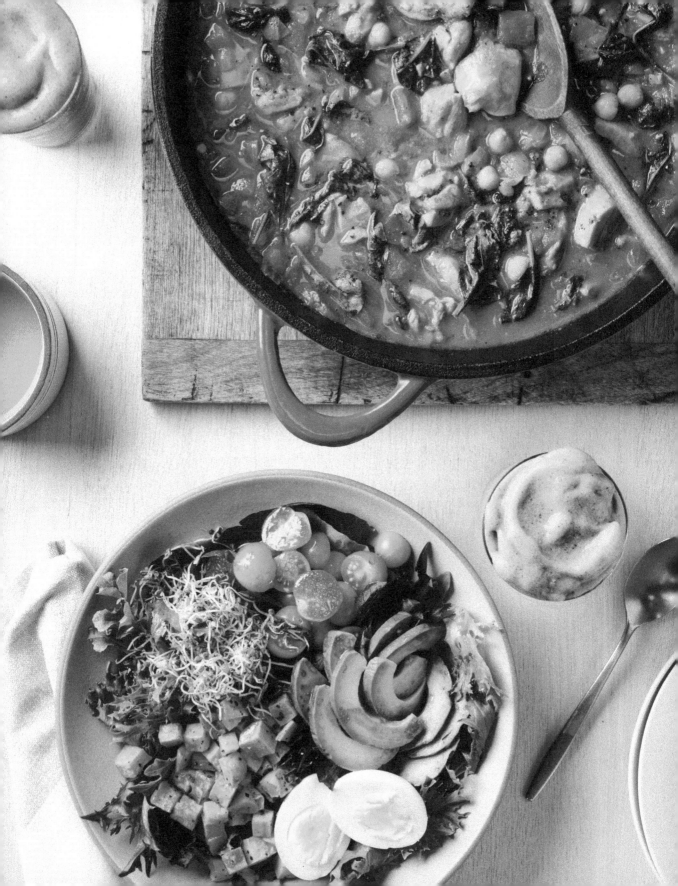

# CONTENTS

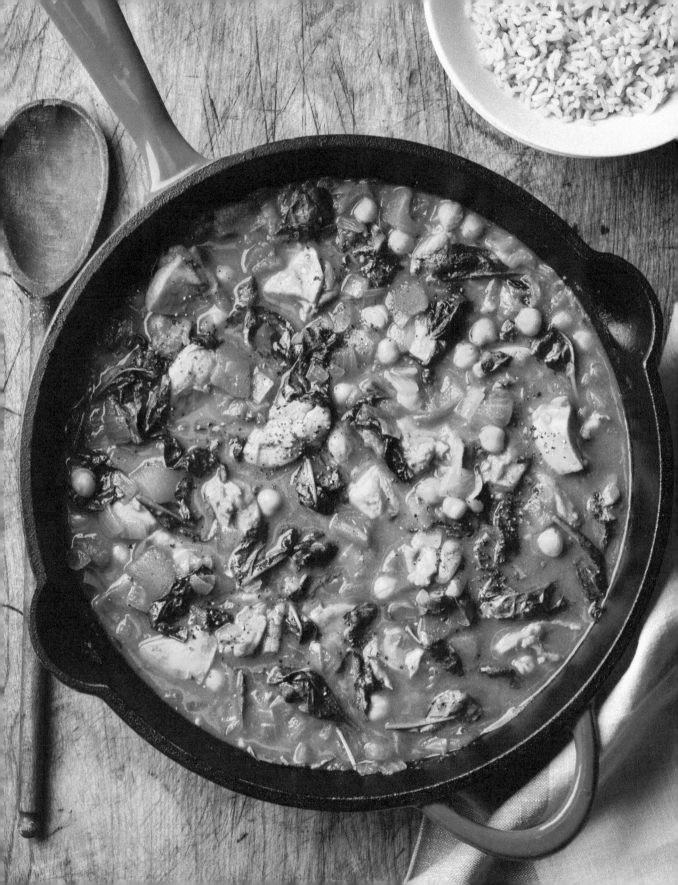

# INTRODUCTION

## When my father was initially diagnosed with cancer, I experienced firsthand the challenges facing cancer patients and their families.

I had been working with cancer patients as a dietitian for several years prior to his diagnosis, and thankfully I was in a position to put all my research and clinical experience to good use.

For the next six months, he went through intensive chemotherapy while following the meal plan we put into place for him. Not only was it effective, but it also helped him move through treatment with very few side effects while still working and living his life.

Not everyone's experience is exactly like my father's, but even so I continue to be amazed at how the right foods and strategies can dramatically impact a person's cancer journey. This is why I've dedicated myself to helping others optimize their cancer recovery, and why I wanted to write this cookbook.

If you've bought this book, then I imagine you're facing a really challenging time right now. Cancer is one of the scariest life-changing experiences we can have—for ourselves and for our loved ones. From the moment you hear that diagnosis, you are on a cancer recovery journey. And in my opinion, the most powerful healing step you can take is to optimize your diet. This information is not readily available and often not being discussed at oncology appointments. And yet it can have a powerful and positive impact on your cancer journey.

In this book you will find easy and tasty recipes to nourish you on your journey. These are recipes that center on healing, cancer-fighting foods. They are recipes that can help minimize the side effects of treatment while giving you the energy and strength to not only move forward but also continue to enjoy your life.

Cancer is one of the most intense, challenging journeys a person can face, yet so much good can come out of it. It is my sincere hope that the information and recipes in this book will not only nourish your body but also empower you to make dietary choices that will fuel your recovery.

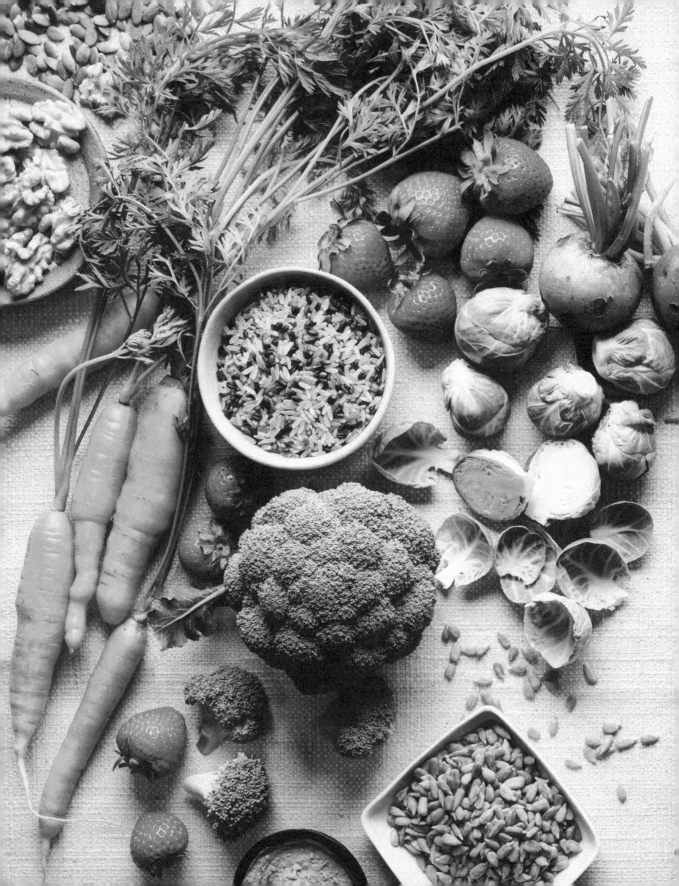

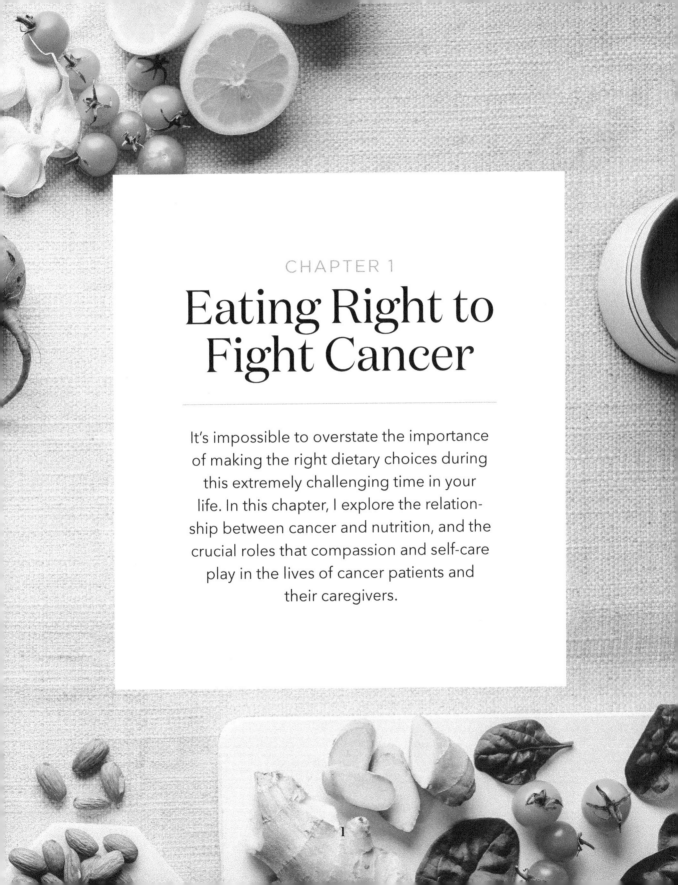

# CHAPTER 1

# Eating Right to Fight Cancer

It's impossible to overstate the importance of making the right dietary choices during this extremely challenging time in your life. In this chapter, I explore the relationship between cancer and nutrition, and the crucial roles that compassion and self-care play in the lives of cancer patients and their caregivers.

## How Cancer Affects the Body

Cancer starts in the cells of the body. Normal cells grow and divide, and they know when to stop. They die when they're supposed to and they reproduce when more cells are needed. Cancer cells, on the other hand, do not behave like normal cells. They continue to grow and divide uncontrollably. They can avoid the immune system and ignore signals that tell them to die or stop growing.

It often takes many years for these cancer cells to grow large enough to form a tumor. A growing tumor can destroy the normal cells around it and begin to damage the body's healthy tissues. Depending on where the tumor is located, it can impact the body in many ways. Sometimes, cancer cells break away from the original tumor and travel to other areas of the body, where they continue to grow and divide and eventually form new tumors at new locations.

Cancer can start almost anywhere in the body. There are more than 100 different types of cancer, and they are generally named for the organs or tissues where they started. Many end up forming solid tumors, but some types, like leukemia or lymphoma, do not. These cancers start in the blood or lymphatic system.

Treatment options depend on the type of cancer that is diagnosed, whether the cancer has spread, and the general health of the patient. The goal of treatment is to kill as many cancerous cells as possible while reducing the damage to normal cells that are nearby.

The most common treatments for cancer include surgery, which directly removes the tumor; chemotherapy, which uses chemicals to kill cancer cells; and radiation, which uses X-rays to kill cancer cells. There are also some cancers that can be treated with immunotherapy, which stimulates the immune system to help the body kill cancer; or hormonal therapy, which slows or stops cancer cells that are stimulated by hormones.

Regardless of your type of cancer or what treatment you are receiving, the healing process can be supported by eating certain foods and avoiding others.

## The Importance of Nutrition During Cancer

Your diet can help you heal in two ways: the foods you eat can help support the treatment while minimizing the side effects, and they can provide you with the energy and strength you need to fuel your recovery. By choosing the right foods, you can have a positive impact on your healing journey. There is no one right diet for everyone, but throughout your cancer journey it's important to make sure you're eating enough calories and protein to maintain your weight, energy, and strength. You should also make sure you're consuming enough micronutrients (vitamins, minerals, and other phytonutrients) to keep your immune system strong and to support the healing process.

## Cancer-Fighting Foods

Adequate protein intake is essential to support energy production, maintain muscle mass, bolster the immune system, and help the body heal and repair. Patients often underestimate how much protein their body needs during cancer treatment. To help you reach your protein goals each day, I suggest including a high-protein food at every meal and every snack. Pasture-raised meats, wild-caught fish, organic dairy products, beans, nuts, seeds, and tofu are all great sources of protein.

Healthy, anti-inflammatory fats—such as oily fish, avocados, nuts, seeds, olive oils, and butter from grass-fed cows—are excellent sources of calories that also nourish the immune system, the nervous system, and all your cellular membranes. Make it a goal to include at least one healthy fat at every meal.

All vegetables can be part of a cancer-healing diet, but when you need to get the most benefit from each bite, I suggest starting with leafy greens, such as kale, spinach, chard, cabbage, or escarole. The wide variety of vitamins, minerals, and phytonutrients in leafy greens support all the necessary systems for healing. Make it a goal to include at least two servings of leafy greens every day; to make this easier, consider that one serving equals 1 cup raw greens or ½ cup cooked.

Alliums—the group of flowering plants that includes garlic, onions, shallots, leeks, and chives—contain compounds that have incredible powers to support detoxification, build immunity, and help the body fight cancer. These vegetables also contain antimicrobial compounds that help fight bacteria, viruses, and other infections when your immune system may be compromised from treatment. Make it a goal to include alliums in at least one meal every day.

And when it comes to fruit, none pack as much healing benefit as berries, which offer an assortment of phytonutrients that can boost the immune system, assist with healing and repair, and help the body fight cancer. Make it a goal to vary your choice of berries and include at least one serving of berries every day.

## Foods to Avoid

Perhaps you have been told to "eat whatever you want, because now is not the time to worry about your diet" or "just eat whatever sounds good, because the most important thing is to keep your weight on." I'm here to tell you that this advice couldn't be further from the truth. If there was ever a time to care about the food you put in your body, now is it.

Some foods are not safe to consume during treatment if your immune system is compromised and you are therefore at a high risk for infections. Be mindful to avoid raw fish, meat, or eggs; unpasteurized dairy products; undercooked meats; and unpasteurized juices (unless you're making them yourself from fresh fruits and veggies). There are also some foods that will be harder to digest during treatment and can cause uncomfortable digestive symptoms, such as fried, greasy, or really spicy foods. And finally, and most important, there are some foods that may actually promote cancer growth, lower your immune response, and work against your healing efforts. These foods include sugar, refined carbohydrates (commonly found in white flour bread, cereal, and pasta), inflammatory fats, processed meats, and meats cooked at really high temperatures (broiling or grilling).

When eating is a challenge and you need to make every bite count, don't waste those bites on food that is not going to be helpful to you.

## THE IMPORTANCE OF TALKING ABOUT SYMPTOMS

As you move through treatment, it's important that you keep your caregivers and care providers in the loop about how you're feeling. If the symptoms are changing or seem to be getting worse, or new ones are appearing, let your care team know about this, as it's possible that different foods or strategies, or even medications, can be introduced to help you feel better. When I work with clients one-on-one, we start every appointment with a review of their symptoms—that's how important it is.

To help you monitor how your symptoms are changing, you might want to consider using a tracking system. Keep a list of important markers, like energy level, digestion, sleep, nausea, pain, or anything else that seems to bother you. At the end of each day, rank the symptoms on a scale from 0 to 5, where 0 means it's not a problem at all and 5 means it's a debilitating problem. As you try different strategies or foods or medications, you can track how each is helping you. Then on the day of your appointment, you can more easily update your providers without needing to rely solely on your memory.

## Taking Control of Your Symptoms Through Diet

In addition to supporting your healing process, certain foods can help improve any symptoms and dramatically impact your overall well-being during your cancer journey. Everyone's experience will be different, owing to the different types of cancer and treatment involved, but here is a guide to some of the more common symptoms people experience and some specific strategies that help minimize these side effects.

### NAUSEA

Nausea is a common side effect of most forms of chemotherapy, as well as radiation that is directed toward the brain, stomach, or abdomen. Thankfully, most people can control their nausea quite well simply by taking the prescribed anti-nausea medications as directed. If this is not enough, however, or if you are not tolerating the medications, starting your morning with a cup of warm ginger tea can be helpful. Many people also find that tart or tangy foods are better tolerated. Eating smaller, more frequent meals also helps, as does avoiding rich, greasy, fried, spicy, or overly sweet foods. Room-temperature foods may be better tolerated than hot or cold ones. And you might even find that not drinking on an empty stomach can be helpful; consider eating a few crackers or a slice of toast before you drink to absorb the extra stomach acid.

Recipes to help with nausea: Morning Tonic, page 146; Stomach-Soothing Juice, page 152; Cinnamon-Spiced Apple Compote with Nut Butter, page 48; Roasted Sweet Potato Fries, page 68.

### FATIGUE

Fatigue, or having very low energy, is another common side effect of almost all types of treatment. In addition to allowing adequate time for sleep and rest, make sure you include a high-protein food at every meal or snack. Also make sure you're eating enough calories, as well as sufficient micronutrients like the B vitamins, iron, or magnesium. I suggest that every meal include at least three parts: protein + fat + colorful plants. Also, avoid skipping meals and make a commitment to eat something every three to four hours; doing so will help ensure you're receiving a continuous supply of energy-supporting nutrients.

Hydration also plays a role in maintaining energy levels, so be sure to include something to drink.

Recipes to help with fatigue: Dark Chocolate Brownie Bites, page 49; Veggie Breakfast Burritos, page 36; Balanced Green Smoothie, page 154; Tuna Pesto Pasta with Broccoli, page 129.

### TROUBLE SWALLOWING

Difficulty in swallowing, also known as dysphagia, is a common side effect for people with mouth or esophageal cancers. Radiation treatment or surgery to this area can also make it painful and difficult to swallow. To help keep both your weight and your nutrition status up, stick with soft and moist foods like smoothies, fresh juices, vegetable purees, scrambled eggs, hummus, bean dips, hot cereals, yogurt, kefir, blended soups, and avocado. You may also need to experiment a bit with the thickness of what you're eating: some foods may be easier to swallow when they are thinned out a bit, like hot cereals, smoothies, scrambled eggs, or purees, while others may need to be thickened a little, like soups, broths, or juices. What's most important when swallowing becomes a challenge is to make every bite count—be mindful of your protein, fat, and nutrient intake. Focusing on smaller, more frequent meals will also make this easier.

Recipes to help with trouble swallowing: Power-Packed Hot Cereal, page 23; Lemon and Rosemary Bean Dip, page 56; Savory Sweet Potato Puree, page 72; Roasted Butternut Squash, Apple, and Sage Soup, page 88.

## ANEMIA

Anemia, a condition that can result from chemotherapy or radiation, occurs when the number of red blood cells drops too low. These are the cells responsible for carrying oxygen throughout the body, and when there are fewer of them, the body has to work harder to get oxygen to all your tissues. This leads to extreme fatigue, shortness of breath, and lightheadedness. If you are experiencing anemia, consuming protein is essential, so every time you eat, even if it's just a snack, be sure to include some protein. Foods rich in iron and the B vitamins will also help; these include meats, poultry, eggs, fish, dark leafy greens, beans, and lentils. Adding foods rich in vitamin C, like berries, citrus, tomatoes, bell pepper, or broccoli, can also help increase the absorption of iron. Try to include foods from these lists at least once or twice a day, and if you're not vegetarian, then get at least one serving of organic grass-fed red meat every week.

Recipes to help with anemia: Spinach and Black Bean Breakfast Bowl, page 43; Spinach Egg Salad, page 62; Harira-Inspired Stew, page 114; Curried Chicken with Chickpeas, page 138.

## TASTE CHANGES

Patients undergoing chemotherapy, radiation to the head or neck, or other medication therapies can often lose their senses of taste or smell, and they may also experience the sensation of food not tasting "right"—that is, seeming bland, metallic, bitter, or too sweet. There are some strategies that "trick" the taste buds, thereby helping make the food more palatable.

For example, try using a mouth rinse before eating to help neutralize the taste buds; just mix a bit of baking soda with some water, then swish and spit it out. To enhance dull or bland flavors, consider adding a pinch of sea salt or a spritz of lemon or lime juice to whatever you're eating. Eating foods loaded with tart flavors—such as pickles, vinegar, or fermented foods—or adding more spice can also help.

To eliminate a metallic taste in your mouth, avoid using metal utensils, cups, or water bottles, and instead try BPA-free plastic, wood, or glass. You can also add a touch of sweetener to cut the metallic taste to whatever you're eating. If food is tasting too salty, add some fresh lemon juice to neutralize the salt. And if food is tasting too sweet, add a few drops of lemon or lime juice.

Recipes to help with taste change: Tomato and Basil Salad, page 76; Moroccan-Spiced Chicken, page 134; Carrot, Beet, and Turmeric Juice, page 150; Lemon-Garlic Dressing, page 168.

## SORE MOUTH OR THROAT

After certain types of chemotherapy or radiation to the head and neck, patients often experience mouth sores or a general sensitivity in the mouth or throat. Soft and moist foods will be more comfortable and easier to eat in these cases. It may also help to avoid highly acidic, spicy, or salty foods, as well as chocolate and caffeine. I also suggest eating foods at room temperature or even a bit chilled. Foods that are cooling and healing, such as avocado, cucumber, mint, coconut oil, raw honey, and aloe vera juice, will not only feel good in the mouth but can also help heal the soreness. You can even try applying a bit of coconut oil or honey to the sores to help soothe them and encourage healing.

Recipes to help with sore mouth or throat: Sweet Potato Porridge, page 34; Spring Green Soup, page 108; Soothing Throat Elixir, page 147; Mineral-Rich Bone Broth, page 160.

## UNINTENTIONAL WEIGHT LOSS

Losing weight can be a serious side effect of cancer treatment that can result in a change in the treatment plan, along with increased fatigue and lower immune response. This can happen for any number of reasons, but usually it's a combination of an increase in nutritional needs and a general lack of appetite. Symptoms such as mouth sores, taste changes, and difficulty swallowing can also make it harder to eat in order to maintain your normal weight.

As a first step, make eating a non-negotiable part of your treatment, even if you don't feel like doing so. Schedule "mini-meals" every two to three hours, and set an alarm to help you remember that it's time to eat. Commit to taking at least a few bites at each mealtime, and make every bite count. Eat your protein first and add foods high in calories that can easily fit with whatever else you're eating so it doesn't feel like just more food—for example, butter or ghee from grass-fed cows, olive oil, avocado oil, coconut oil, full-fat coconut milk, nut or seed butters, or whole-fat dairy foods. You may also want to add an unflavored, organic whey protein powder that you can easily mix into whatever else you're eating. Mild exercise will also help stimulate your appetite and preserve muscle mass.

Recipes to help with unintentional weight loss: Nourishing High-Calorie Smoothie, page 155; Lemon-Herb Chicken Salad, page 64; Avocado Tuna Boats, page 61; Almond Butter and Banana Toast, page 22.

## DIARRHEA

Digestive changes, including diarrhea, are common side effects of chemotherapy and radiation or surgery in the abdominal area. Diarrhea can lead to dehydration, weight loss, and fatigue if left untreated. Your doctor may suggest medications to help manage the diarrhea, but no matter what, make sure you are drinking a lot of fluids to prevent dehydration. Fluids with electrolytes in them are even better, like broths, soups, fresh vegetable juices, or coconut water. Limit or avoid milk and other dairy foods, sugar-sweetened beverages, foods or drinks sweetened with sugar alcohols, and fried or greasy foods. And to minimize the diarrhea, eat more foods high in *soluble* fiber, like oatmeal, oat bran, lentils, apples, oranges, pears, strawberries, nuts, flaxseed, beans, dried peas, blueberries, psyllium, or bananas. Also consider adding more probiotic-rich foods to your meals, like miso, sauerkraut, kefir, pickles, or tempeh.

Recipes to help with diarrhea: Berry Baked Oatmeal, page 24; Blueberry Flax Muffins, page 32; Black Bean–Stuffed Sweet Potatoes, page 120; French Lentil Salad, page 84.

## CONSTIPATION

Constipation is a common digestive change that can occur as a result of treatment or even as a side effect of certain medications, like anti-nausea prescriptions. Adequate hydration is important here. Keep track of how much you're typically drinking and make it a goal to increase this by another 2 to 4 cups a day. Warm and hot fluids can help stimulate a bowel movement. Warm prune juice is remarkably effective, as are many different herbal teas, and even fresh veggie juice can help.

To help alleviate constipation, increase your intake of foods high in *insoluble* fiber, like whole wheat or other whole grains, seeds, nuts, broccoli, cabbage, onions, dark leafy vegetables, raisins, grapes, or other fresh or dried fruits. Be careful to not overdo the vegetables that increase gas production, like broccoli and cabbage, and avoid carbonated beverages, as these can sometimes make your symptoms more uncomfortable. Adding more healthy fats and oils to your food can also help stimulate movement in your gut. You might try adding a spoonful of coconut oil to a cup of warm tea first thing in the morning.

Recipes to help with constipation: Zesty Green Juice, page 151; Green Tea Detox, page 148; Kale Salad, page 74; Homemade Granola, page 26.

## FOODS THAT HELP YOU HEAL

| FOOD | CANCER-FIGHTING PROPERTIES | TARGET SYMPTOMS | HEALING RECIPES |
|---|---|---|---|
| Avocado | Good source of fiber & healthy fat<br><br>Healthy calories<br><br>Anti-inflammatory | Fatigue<br><br>Sore mouth/throat<br><br>Trouble swallowing<br><br>Weight loss | Green Pea Guacamole (page 55)<br><br>Avocado Tuna Boats (page 61) |
| Beans | Good source of fiber, iron, B vitamins & protein<br><br>Supports digestion | Anemia<br><br>Diarrhea<br><br>Fatigue<br><br>Trouble swallowing | Curry Hummus (page 54)<br><br>Turkey and Bean Chili (page 140) |

| FOOD | CANCER-FIGHTING PROPERTIES | TARGET SYMPTOMS | HEALING RECIPES |
|---|---|---|---|
| Beets | Good source of B vitamins, iron, vitamin C & fiber<br><br>Detox supporting<br><br>Anti-inflammatory | Anemia<br><br>Constipation<br><br>Fatigue | Warm Beet, Feta, and Mint Salad (page 78)<br><br>Carrot, Beet, and Turmeric Juice (page 150) |
| Berries | Good source of vitamin C, fiber & antioxidants<br><br>Anti-inflammatory<br><br>Immune boosting | Anemia<br><br>Diarrhea<br><br>Nausea<br><br>Taste changes | Berry Baked Oatmeal (page 24)<br><br>Anticancer Rainbow Smoothie (page 153) |
| Brazil nuts | Good source of selenium, fiber & healthy fats<br><br>Healthy calories<br><br>Supports digestion<br><br>Anti-inflammatory | Constipation<br><br>Diarrhea<br><br>Fatigue<br><br>Weight loss | Homemade Granola (page 26)<br><br>Healthy Trail Mix (page 51) |
| Broccoli (& other cruciferous veggies) | Good source of fiber, B vitamins, vitamin C, antioxidants & phytonutrients<br><br>Detox supporting<br><br>Hormone balancing<br><br>Antibacterial against *H. pylori* | Anemia<br><br>Constipation<br><br>Fatigue | Rainbow Slaw (page 75)<br><br>Golden Cauliflower (page 69) |
| Carrots | Good source of vitamin A, carotenoids, fiber & phytonutrients<br><br>Immune boosting<br><br>Anti-inflammatory<br><br>Detox supporting | Diarrhea<br><br>Fatigue | Carrot, Apple, and Walnut Muffins (page 52)<br><br>Carrot, Beet, and Turmeric Juice (page 150) |

*continues*

| FOOD | CANCER-FIGHTING PROPERTIES | TARGET SYMPTOMS | HEALING RECIPES |
|---|---|---|---|
| Celery | Good source of vitamin C, potassium & antioxidants<br><br>Anti-inflammatory<br><br>Supports digestion | Diarrhea<br><br>Fatigue | Zesty Green Juice (page 151)<br><br>Stomach-Soothing Juice (page 152) |
| Citrus | Good source of vitamin C, fiber & antioxidants<br><br>Immune boosting<br><br>Detox supporting | Diarrhea<br><br>Nausea<br><br>Taste changes | Herbal Citrus Marinade (page 174)<br><br>Lemon-Garlic Dressing (page 168) |
| Flaxseed (& other seeds) | Good source of fiber, healthy fats & phytonutrients<br><br>Healthy calories<br><br>Hormone balancing<br><br>Supports digestion | Diarrhea<br><br>Fatigue<br><br>Weight loss | Blueberry Flax Muffins (page 32)<br><br>Homemade Granola (page 26) |
| Garlic (& other alliums) | Good source of sulfur compounds & other phytonutrients<br><br>Antimicrobial<br><br>Immune boosting<br><br>Detox supporting<br><br>Supports digestion | Constipation<br><br>Taste changes | Garlic-Herb Yogurt Dip (page 58)<br><br>Balsamic Vinaigrette (page 167) |
| Ginger | Good source of various vitamins, minerals & phytonutrients<br><br>Supports digestion<br><br>Anti-inflammatory<br><br>Antimicrobial<br><br>Immune boosting | Constipation<br><br>Diarrhea<br><br>Nausea<br><br>Taste changes | Morning Tonic (page 146)<br><br>Curried Chicken with Chickpeas (page 138) |

| FOOD | CANCER-FIGHTING PROPERTIES | TARGET SYMPTOMS | HEALING RECIPES |
|---|---|---|---|
| Green Tea | Good source of antioxidants & catechins (especially EGCG)<br><br>Detox supporting<br><br>Anti-inflammatory<br><br>Immune boosting | Sore mouth/throat<br><br>Taste changes<br><br>Trouble swallowing | Green Tea Detox (page 148) |
| Mushrooms | Good source of antioxidants, B vitamins, vitamin D & beta-glucan fiber<br><br>Immune boosting<br><br>Anti-inflammatory<br><br>Supports digestion<br><br>Hormone balancing | Anemia<br><br>Constipation<br><br>Diarrhea<br><br>Fatigue | Mushroom Burgers (page 125)<br><br>Mushroom Barley Soup (page 98) |
| Salmon (& other oily fish) | Good source of protein, vitamin $B_{12}$, zinc, antioxidants & healthy fats<br><br>Healthy calories<br><br>Anti-inflammatory | Anemia<br><br>Fatigue<br><br>Sore mouth/throat<br><br>Weight loss | Baked Salmon with Asparagus, Tomatoes, and Potatoes (page 126)<br><br>Easy Lemon-Butter Fish (page 128) |
| Spinach (& other leafy greens) | Good source of iron, B vitamins, carotenoids & phytonutrients<br><br>Immune boosting<br><br>Anti-inflammatory<br><br>Detox supporting | Anemia<br><br>Constipation<br><br>Fatigue | Kale Salad (page 72)<br><br>Basil-Spinach Pesto (page 172)<br><br>Simple Sautéed Greens (page 71) |

*continues*

| FOOD | CANCER-FIGHTING PROPERTIES | TARGET SYMPTOMS | HEALING RECIPES |
|---|---|---|---|
| Tofu (& other whole soy foods) | Good source of protein, iron, calcium & isoflavones<br><br>Hormone balancing | Anemia<br><br>Fatigue<br><br>Sore mouth/throat<br><br>Trouble swallowing | Tofu and Mushroom Stir-Fry with Bok Choy (page 122)<br><br>Miso Soup with Tofu and Greens (page 102) |
| Tomatoes | Good source of vitamin C, potassium, lycopene & other phytonutrients<br><br>Anti-inflammatory<br><br>Supports digestion | Anemia<br><br>Constipation<br><br>Fatigue<br><br>Taste changes | Tomato and Basil Salad (page 76)<br><br>Spaghetti with Mushroom Bolognese (page 118) |
| Turmeric | Good source of manganese, iron & phytonutrients (especially curcumin)<br><br>Anti-inflammatory<br><br>Detox supporting<br><br>Immune boosting<br><br>Antimicrobial | Constipation<br><br>Diarrhea<br><br>Nausea<br><br>Taste changes | Turmeric Scrambled Eggs (page 38)<br><br>Turmeric Milk (page 149)<br><br>Creamy Turmeric Dressing (page 170) |
| Walnuts (& other nuts) | Good source of protein, fiber, vitamin E & healthy fats<br><br>Healthy calories<br><br>Anti-inflammatory<br><br>Supports digestion | Constipation<br><br>Diarrhea<br><br>Fatigue<br><br>Weight loss | Walnut Chicken with Pomegranate (page 142)<br><br>Walnut, Pear, and Pomegranate Salad (page 77) |

# Self-Care for Caregivers

Caregivers are the unsung heroes of the cancer journey. In my work with cancer patients, I am continually checking in with their caregivers to make sure they have the support they need to take care of themselves. With that in mind, here are some tips to help make life a little easier for caregivers:

- Whenever possible, batch-cook meals to have leftovers or store extra servings in the freezer for a later date.

- Recruit other family members and friends to help cook and prepare meals; now is not the time to shy away from outside support. Share your favorite recipes with them so they know what to cook for you.

- If your budget allows, consider grocery or healthy meal delivery options to reduce your workload.

- Much as we recommend for mothers with newborn babies, when the person with cancer is resting, take some time for yourself. Take a nap, do something fun, get in a little exercise, lie in the sun, read a book, take a hot bath, do some meditation, or anything else that would be restorative and nourishing for you. This is how you build resilience.

- Laugh every day! Yep, you read that right. Actually, this is an excellent tip for the person with cancer, as well. Watch a funny movie or comedy routine, tell jokes, call a friend who always makes you laugh. Laughter is medicine. It reduces stress, boosts the immune system, supports healing, is energizing, and will help you get through this.

## What to Eat Before Treatment

There is a lot you can do in the weeks leading up to treatment that will better prepare you to have a successful cancer journey. Now is the time to build up your reserves; it's your opportunity to optimize your diet and nourish your body with all the nutrients it's going to need to help you heal and recover.

If you are not already doing so, get into the habit of eating three meals each day—meals that are balanced with protein, healthy fats, colorful plants, and low-glycemic carbohydrates. Make it a goal to consume as many fresh vegetables and fruits as possible. Slowly start weaning yourself off the foods that can interfere with healing, like sugars, refined carbohydrates, soda/other sweetened beverages, fried foods, fast food, processed meats, and alcohol. In between your meals, drink more water, green tea, herbal tea, or fresh veggie juice.

Take the time to batch-cook some meals and stock your freezer with healing, cancer-fighting, strengthening meals that you can pull out during your treatment time when you don't feel like cooking. Along these same lines, stock your pantry with staples that you can turn to for quick, nourishing meals or snacks.

Many of the recipes in this book lend themselves well to batch-cooking. Here are some you can make in the weeks leading up to treatment: Mineral-Rich Bone Broth (or any of the other broth recipes), page 160; Turkey and Bean Chili, page 140; Harira-Inspired Stew, page 114; Veggie Breakfast Burritos, page 36.

## What to Eat During Treatment

Once treatment has started, there are some strategies you can use to help minimize any side effects and support your healing, one of which is to not eat at all. You may be asked to fast before surgery, but you can also use fasting to help you better tolerate the chemotherapy and radiation. Studies have shown that fasting during cancer treatment is safe and may help protect healthy cells while making the cancer cells more vulnerable to treatment. We also know that fasting lowers inflammation and blood sugar levels, both of which can help support healing and lessen the symptoms caused by treatment.

But there are some instances when fasting is not recommended. For patients who are already underweight or malnourished, or at high risk for cachexia ("wasting" disorder), it's best to not add fasting to your protocol. For those with diabetes or other chronic health diseases, fasting may also not be recommended. As with any integrative cancer strategy, you should work with your provider to make sure your methods are appropriate and safe for you to follow.

If you want to try fasting, start with an overnight fast of at least 12 to 14 hours during each night of the weeks preceding treatment. This alone has been shown to help boost the immune system, support healing, and reduce cancer risk. Once this nighttime fasting feels easy to do, you can then try extending the fast to 16 to 18 hours several times a week, either by eating dinner earlier or having breakfast later, or a combination of the two.

If having radiation, once your treatment begins, you can try to fast 14 hours just prior to treatment and then wait another 1 to 2 hours afterward before you eat. Admittedly, this will be much easier to do if your radiation treatments are in the morning. If having chemotherapy, you can try to eat your dinner as early as possible the night before treatment, and then fast the entire day of treatment, focusing on drinking fluids instead. For example, make it a goal to drink 8 to 10 ounces of liquid every hour that you are awake. You can vary it between water, green tea, herbal tea, or broth. Then, if you can, continue the fast until the following day's breakfast or lunch. Most people are not very hungry the day of treatment and find it easier than they expected to fast this way. There are some scenarios where it could be helpful to fast longer, but do this only under the guidance of your provider, especially if your chemotherapy requires multiple days of treatment.

If you decide not to fast or you determine that this would not be safe for you, then include light foods that do not require too much digestive energy on the days of treatment. Soups, broths, smoothies, and fresh juices would all be great options. Focusing on fluids is the most important strategy you can apply on the days of treatment and the first few days after.

Recipes that would work well on treatment day: Mineral-Rich Bone Broth, page 160; Green Tea Detox, page 148; Healthy Trail Mix (in case you get hungry and need to break your fast or if you're not fasting), page 51.

## What to Eat After Treatment

In between treatment days, it is important to continue to focus on fluids and protein, as your needs for both are higher than normal. Protein is probably the biggest influence on how you feel, as it will keep up your energy and strength while also supporting your healing and your immune system. Depending on what symptoms arise from treatment, you can refer to the suggestions outlined earlier for some of the more common side effects and create a food plan that works best for you.

Once treatment is over, your symptoms can persist for a few weeks to a few months. In the first four to six weeks following treatment, focus on rebuilding and replenishing your reserves; take advantage of your gradually improving appetite. There is still a lot of detoxification, healing, and repair that is happening, and you can best support these processes by focusing on high-quality nutrition, adequate hydration, plenty of sleep and rest, and daily exercise.

Recipes to consider post-treatment: Herb-Roasted Chicken and Potatoes, page 130; Walnut Chicken with Pomegranate, page 142; Veggie Frittata, page 124.

## THE ROLE OF SELF-COMPASSION

In your quest to optimize your diet and eat more healing foods, there is some wiggle room—it's what I call the "80/20 Rule." That is, what you do 80 percent of the time will have the biggest impact on your health and healing. So, if you are filling that 80 percent with all the foods and meals and strategies described in this book, then guess what? There is room to splurge—20 percent, to be exact. Maybe that means allowing yourself a slice of your favorite chocolate cake on your birthday, or having a special meal at a restaurant when you reach the halfway point, or sipping a glass of Champagne to celebrate a good scan.

You get the point. Life is meant to be lived, enjoyed, and celebrated, and just because you are currently dealing with cancer doesn't mean you can't still live and enjoy life. It also does not mean that the occasional treat or splurge will completely negate your efforts. You can do this. I know you can, because I've seen many other people get through this. Things do not have to be perfect all the time for you to be moving in the right direction. Put one foot in front of the other, and keep going.

## Kitchen Staples

The recipes in this book use commonly available foods that you should be able to find at any grocery store. Organic ingredients are worth seeking out, as they will boost the nutritional quality of your diet and limit your exposure to pesticides and other chemicals. It's also a good idea to stick with real, whole foods whenever possible. Some quality frozen, jarred, and canned goods are nice to have on hand, too. Here are some staples that will help you make the nutritious meals in this book:

**Healthy Oils:** extra-virgin olive oil, coconut oil, avocado oil, and butter or ghee from grass-fed cows

**Condiments:** balsamic vinegar, apple cider vinegar, Dijon mustard, tomato sauce, canned diced tomatoes, miso paste, pickles and/or sauerkraut

**Nondairy Milks:** unsweetened coconut milk and almond milk

**Sweeteners:** honey, maple syrup, dates and other dried fruits, dark chocolate or cocoa powder (ideally 70 percent or higher)

**Starches:** rice (brown, wild, white), oats, quinoa, whole-grain or bean-based pasta, whole-grain or sprouted bread, corn tortillas, and other whole-grain products you enjoy

**Proteins:** beans (chickpea, black, kidney, white, etc.), lentils, raw nuts (almonds, walnuts, pistachios, cashews, etc.), raw seeds (pumpkin, flax, chia, etc.), nut butters (peanut, almond, cashew, walnut, etc.), canned fish (tuna, salmon, sardines)

**Frozen Foods:** berries, peas, and other veggies you like

**Fresh Seasonings:** onions, garlic, fresh ginger, fresh turmeric

**Dried Herbs and Spices:** sea salt, black peppercorns, ground turmeric, ground cumin, curry powder, ground ginger, ground cinnamon, herbes de Provence, etc.; the more variety, the better

## Essential Kitchen Equipment

The recipes in this book do not require a lot of equipment, but some key utensils and cookware are necessary and will make it much easier and more enjoyable for you to cook.

**Sharp Knife:** The sharper your knife is, the easier it will be to chop and prep your meals quickly.

**Cutting Boards:** Have at least two cutting boards, one for raw meat, poultry, or fish, and the other for veggies. This will improve food safety and reduce your risk for infection.

**Dutch Oven:** This is essential for making soups, stews, broths, pasta, roasted chicken, and even bread.

**Stainless-Steel Pans/Pots (with lids):** With a properly oiled stainless-steel saucepan or skillet you can cook fish, veggies, omelets, frittatas, or anything else you would normally make in a nonstick pan. It is time to let go of the nonstick pans: they contain harmful chemicals that you don't want leaching into your food. A well-seasoned cast-iron skillet or an enamel-coated saucepan also works well.

**Baking Sheet:** Also known as a sheet pan, this versatile cookware is great for baking and essential for roasting veggies.

**High-Speed Blender:** The extra power offered by these blenders is best for making everything from smoothies to salad dressings.

**Food Processor:** A time-saver, the food processor can chop vegetables, puree soups, and blend sauces and dressings.

**Glass Storage Containers (with lids):** These are essential for storing leftovers, smoothies, juices, dressings, or sauces, and much safer than plastic containers. Mason canning jars work really well and are often less expensive.

## Nice-to-Haves

**Garlic Press, Juice Press, and Zester:** These gadgets are not essential but will save time and make cooking easier.

**Immersion Blender:** It's a lot easier to simply submerge an immersion blender into a large pot of soup or vegetables to puree than to transfer to a blender and puree in batches.

**Electric Pressure Cooker:** This appliance saves time when cooking broths and some soups and makes grains and legumes quickly and easily; the 6-quart capacity is the most practical.

## The Recipes in This Book

The recipes in this book are designed to provide nourishment to cancer patients while also helping alleviate the symptoms associated with treatment. To make things as simple as possible for both patients and caregivers, these recipes are labeled in one of three "easy" categories: (1) they can be made with five or fewer ingredients (other than salt, pepper, olive oil, or water);

(2) they can be cooked in 30 minutes or less from start to finish; or (3) they can be made in one pot, pan, or baking sheet. There are also labels for recipes that are vegetarian or vegan.

**5** 5 Ingredients or Fewer

**30** Under 30 Minutes

**OP** One Pot

**VG** Vegetarian

**V** Vegan

Each recipe also includes dietary information and a listing of symptoms that the dish can help alleviate (also see the recipe index by symptom on page 8). When the recipe yield is a range (such as "Serves 4 to 6"), the nutritional information per serving is based on the first option—that is, the serving size for one portion of four servings prepared, rather than six. Similarly, if an ingredient is presented as a choice of two or more items, the first listed is what was counted in the dietary information. Lastly, optional ingredients are not included in the nutritional totals.

The information in this book is designed to help you build your own meal plans or simply select a healing dish any time you want. It is my sincere hope that these recipes will help you feel better while also providing some nourishing comfort during your cancer journey.

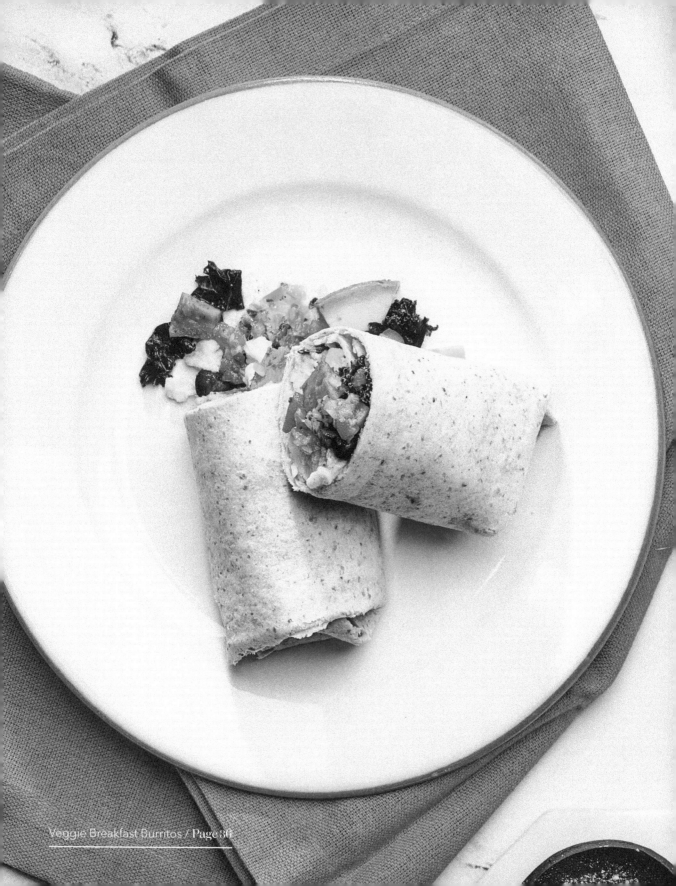

# CHAPTER 2

# Breakfast

# Almond Butter and Banana Toast

SERVES: 2 | PREP TIME: 10 Minutes

SYMPTOMS: Nausea / Fatigue / Unintentional Weight Loss / Diarrhea

2 tablespoons raw
almond butter
2 slices whole-grain or
gluten-free bread, toasted
1 banana, sliced into coins
1 tablespoons chia seeds

When you're not very hungry or nothing sounds good to eat, toast can hit the spot. Almond butter and chia seeds provide the protein and healthy fats your body needs during cancer treatment. You can add a bit of raw honey or a sprinkle of ground cinnamon for extra sweetness. If you're looking for a calorie boost, increase the amount of almond butter or chia seeds, or add a layer of coconut oil before the almond butter.

Spread the almond butter on each slice of toast, top with the banana slices and chia seeds, and serve.

VARIATION TIP: If you're avoiding grains, substitute sweet potato for the toast in this or any other toast recipe. Cut a sweet potato into ½-inch lengthwise slices and bake at 400°F until soft and tender, about 20 minutes. Store in an airtight container in the refrigerator for up to 1 week. When you're ready to make your "toast," simply heat in the toaster oven.

PER SERVING: Calories: 254; Total fat: 12g; Sodium: 102mg; Carbohydrates: 31g; Fiber: 8g; Protein: 9g

# Power-Packed Hot Cereal

30

OP

V

| SERVES: 2 | PREP TIME: 5 Minutes | COOK TIME: 15 Minutes |
|---|---|---|

SYMPTOMS: Nausea / Fatigue / Trouble Swallowing / Taste Changes / Sore Mouth or Throat / Unintentional Weight Loss

½ cup old-fashioned rolled oats

1 cup unsweetened oat milk or almond milk

1 cup berries (such as blueberries), fresh or frozen

½ teaspoon ground cinnamon

Pinch sea salt

2 tablespoons raw almond butter

2 tablespoons ground flaxseed

Chopped walnuts, sliced almonds, sliced fresh fruit, honey, or maple syrup, for topping (optional)

This amped-up oatmeal supplies the protein, healthy fats, antioxidants, and phytonutrients to help fuel your recovery. Oats, berries, and flaxseed are also great sources of soluble fiber, which helps with diarrhea and an upset stomach. This recipe is adaptable, so feel free to use whichever berries you like or happen to have on hand.

1. In a medium saucepan, combine the oats, milk, berries, cinnamon, and salt and bring to a boil over medium-high heat. Cover, reduce the heat to low, and simmer until the liquid is absorbed, about 10 minutes.

2. Remove from the heat, stir, and divide into 2 bowls. Top each bowl with 1 tablespoon of almond butter and 1 tablespoon of flaxseed, plus the toppings, if using.

3. Serve. Store leftovers in an airtight container in the refrigerator for up to 6 days.

PER SERVING: Calories: 310; Total fat: 15g; Sodium: 118mg; Carbohydrates: 37g; Fiber: 9g; Protein: 10g

OP

VG

# Berry Baked Oatmeal

| SERVES: 4 | PREP TIME: 10 Minutes | COOK TIME: 30 Minutes |

SYMPTOMS: Nausea / Fatigue / Taste Changes / Diarrhea

1 cup old-fashioned
  rolled oats

½ cup chopped
  walnuts, divided

½ teaspoon baking powder

1 teaspoon ground cinnamon

Pinch sea salt

1 tablespoon unsalted butter
  (preferably grass-fed),
  melted, plus more
  for greasing

1 cup unsweetened oat milk,
  almond milk, or coconut milk

1 large egg

¼ cup maple syrup

1 teaspoon vanilla extract

2 bananas, sliced into coins

1 cup berries (such as
  strawberries, blueber-
  ries, or mixed), fresh or
  frozen, divided

Baking the oatmeal makes this breakfast staple feel like more of a treat. It's also a well-balanced meal, with plenty of fiber, protein, and healthy fat. The berries and cinnamon provide an antioxidant-packed immune system boost, and the oats, walnuts, and banana support digestion and help ease diarrhea or an upset stomach. To keep the recipe dairy-free, you can substitute coconut oil for the butter. You can also experiment with different nuts; Brazil nuts, pecans, or almonds would also work really well.

1. Preheat the oven to 375°F. Lightly butter a 2-quart baking dish.

2. In a medium bowl, whisk together the oats, ¼ cup of the walnuts, the baking powder, cinnamon, and salt.

3. In a small bowl, whisk together the melted butter, milk, egg, maple syrup, and vanilla.

4. Spread the sliced bananas in a single layer in the bottom of the baking dish. Top with ½ cup of the berries. Sprinkle the oat mixture evenly over the fruit. Pour the butter mixture evenly over the top. Sprinkle with the remaining ¼ cup of walnuts and ½ cup of berries. Bake for 30 minutes, or until the top is browned and the oats have set.

5. Cool for 5 minutes before serving. Serve warm, spooned into bowls. Store leftovers in an airtight container in the refrigerator for up to 6 days or in the freezer for up to 6 months.

PREP AHEAD TIP: This recipe can be made on Sunday and enjoyed over the course of the week. It reheats nicely on the stovetop or in the microwave.

PER SERVING: Calories: 390; Total fat: 16g; Sodium: 72mg; Carbohydrates: 55g; Fiber: 7g; Protein: 9g

# Homemade Granola

SERVES: 6 | PREP TIME: 10 Minutes

SYMPTOMS: Nausea / Fatigue / Unintentional Weight Loss / Diarrhea / Constipation

1 cup raw pumpkin seeds

½ cup raw almonds

½ cup raw walnuts

¼ cup hemp seeds

1 cup unsweetened shredded coconut

½ cup raw almond butter

6 large dates, pitted

½ teaspoon sea salt

½ teaspoon ground cinnamon

VARIATION TIPS: You can tailor the ingredients in this granola to suit your taste. Instead of cinnamon, try ground cardamom, ground ginger, or vanilla extract. You might also consider adding dark chocolate chips or a variety of dried fruits, such as cranberries, apricots, or cherries. The possibilities are endless.

A bowl of cereal can be a comforting option when you don't feel like cooking or nothing else sounds good. This no-cook granola is a quick, healthy alternative to not-so-wholesome boxed cereals. I like to serve it on top of plain yogurt with fresh fruit or with unsweetened almond milk. You can also enjoy it on its own as a snack, or over some sliced bananas with more almond butter. Although roasted nuts and seeds still provide health benefits, I suggest using raw nuts and seeds to avoid added salt, vegetable oil, and other compounds like acrylamide, which can form during roasting. The roasting process can also damage or oxidize the delicate oils in nuts and seeds and may also reduce their antioxidant content.

Put all the ingredients in a food processor. Pulse on and off a few times until the ingredients are combined, then process until the mixture is crumbly, about 2 minutes. Store in an airtight container in the refrigerator for up to 2 weeks.

PER SERVING: Calories: 466; Total fat: 40g; Sodium: 164mg; Carbohydrates: 19g; Fiber: 8g; Protein: 16g

# Chocolate–Peanut Butter Overnight Oats

SERVES: 2

PREP TIME: 5 Minutes

**SYMPTOMS:** Nausea / Fatigue / Trouble Swallowing / Taste Changes / Sore Mouth or Throat / Unintentional Weight Loss / Diarrhea

1 cup old-fashioned rolled oats

1 cup unsweetened oat milk or almond milk

2 tablespoons chia seeds

2 tablespoons natural peanut butter

2 tablespoons dark chocolate chips (70% cacao or higher)

These overnight oats will satisfy your sweet tooth while still providing nourishing calories from protein and healthy fats. Sweet flavors, such as chocolate, are generally well tolerated when you're experiencing taste or appetite changes, and dark chocolate is also a great source of antioxidants and anti-inflammatory phytonutrients. The oats and chia seeds are soothing to the gut and can help ease diarrhea or an upset stomach. You may want to experiment with different fruits, nut butters, seeds, or spices. Some of my favorite variations include banana-walnut, cinnamon-apple, and blueberry.

1. Divide the ingredients evenly between 2 pint-size mason jars or other lidded glass containers. Stir well, making sure the oats are immersed in liquid. Refrigerate overnight.

2. The next morning, open a jar, stir, and eat it cold, or warm through in a saucepan over medium heat. Store the other jar in the refrigerator for up to 5 days.

PER SERVING: Calories: 444; Total fat: 20g; Sodium: 80mg; Carbohydrates: 52g; Fiber: 11g; Protein: 17g

# Plantain Pancakes with Berry Compote

| MAKES: 6 Large Pancakes | PREP TIME: 10 Minutes | COOK TIME: 20 Minutes |
| --- | --- | --- |

SYMPTOMS: Nausea / Taste Changes / Diarrhea

**FOR THE COMPOTE**

2 cups berries (such as blueberries, raspberries, blackberries, or mixed), fresh or frozen

¼ cup maple syrup

2 teaspoons freshly squeezed lemon juice

3 tablespoons water

**FOR THE PANCAKES**

2 large green plantains, quartered and peeled

4 large eggs

2 teaspoons vanilla extract

½ teaspoon baking soda

¼ teaspoon sea salt

1 to 3 tablespoons coconut oil

When you're trying to eat fewer carbohydrates but still craving a morning pancake, this is the recipe to make. The plantains provide all the starch, so there's no flour necessary. They're not quite as fluffy as traditional pancakes, but surprisingly close and just as yummy. The plantains and berries are also great sources of fiber and help support a healthy gut. You can use less maple syrup or no sweetener at all if you prefer a tart berry compote.

1. **To make the compote:** In a small saucepan, bring the berries, maple syrup, lemon juice, and water to a simmer over medium heat. Cook for about 10 minutes, until the berries are soft, then reduce the heat to low. Using a wooden spoon, mash the berries. Cook for another 10 minutes, occasionally mashing the fruit some more to combine.

2. **Meanwhile, make the pancakes:** Place the plantains in a blender or food processor with the eggs, vanilla, baking soda, and salt. Blend until you achieve a smooth batter, 1 to 2 minutes.

3. Melt 1 tablespoon of the coconut oil in a large skillet over medium heat. When the oil is shimmering, pour ½ cup of the batter into the pan and repeat, fitting as many pancakes as you can in the pan without crowding.

4. Cook until the edges of the pancakes are golden brown and bubbles appear on top. Flip the pancakes and cook on the other side for 1 to 2 minutes, until the pancakes are cooked through. Repeat with the remaining batter, adding more coconut oil to your pan as needed. Serve the pancakes topped with warm berry compote.

PER SERVING (1 PANCAKE): Calories: 246; Total fat: 10g; Sodium: 234mg; Carbohydrates: 36g; Fiber: 6g; Protein: 5g

# Healthy Whole-Grain Pancakes

**MAKES: 8 Pancakes** | **PREP TIME: 10 Minutes** | **COOK TIME: 15 Minutes**

**SYMPTOMS:** Nausea / Taste Changes / Sore Mouth or Throat / Unintentional Weight Loss

1½ cups whole wheat or gluten-free flour (such as coconut, almond, or chickpea flour)

½ teaspoon sea salt

1 tablespoon plus 1 teaspoon baking powder

1 cup organic whole milk

1 large egg

2 tablespoons unsalted butter (preferably grass-fed), melted, plus more for greasing

Raw honey, maple syrup, berry compote, fresh fruit, or nut butter, for topping (optional)

By using whole-grain, bean, or nut-based flours in these pancakes, you are increasing the fiber content and lowering the glycemic load, without sacrificing flavor. The milk, butter, and egg add healthy calories and protein, but you can easily substitute unsweetened almond or coconut milk for the milk, and coconut or avocado oil for the butter to make these dairy-free.

1. In a large bowl, whisk the flour, salt, and baking powder to combine.

2. In a medium bowl, whisk the milk and egg to combine.

3. Create a well in the center of the flour mixture. Pour in the melted butter and the egg mixture. Whisk until just combined, taking care not to overmix. The batter should be slightly thick and lumpy. Let the batter rest for 5 to 10 minutes; this will make fluffier pancakes.

4. Using a paper towel dabbed with some melted butter, lightly grease a large skillet. Heat the skillet over medium heat until hot. Drizzle a drop of water onto the surface; if it sizzles, the skillet is ready.

5. Pour ⅓ cup of the batter into the skillet and repeat, fitting in as many pancakes as you can without crowding.

6. Cook until the bottom edges of the pancakes are golden brown and bubbles appear on top, then flip the pancakes and cook the other side for 1 to 2 minutes, until the pancakes are cooked through. Repeat with the remaining batter, adding more melted butter as needed. Serve warm with your favorite toppings, if desired.

PER SERVING (2 PANCAKES): Calories: 264; Total fat: 10g; Sodium: 283mg; Carbohydrates: 38g; Fiber: 5g; Protein: 10g

# Blueberry Flax Muffins

| MAKES: **12 Muffins** | PREP TIME: **10 Minutes** | COOK TIME: **30 Minutes** |

SYMPTOMS: Nausea / Fatigue / Sore Mouth or Throat / Unintentional Weight Loss / Diarrhea

2 cups whole wheat or
  gluten-free flour (such
  as coconut, almond, or
  chickpea flour)
½ cup ground flaxseed
½ cup brown sugar
1 teaspoon baking powder
1 teaspoon ground cinnamon
1 teaspoon ground nutmeg
½ teaspoon sea salt
2 cups blueberries, fresh
  or frozen
2 large eggs
½ cup organic whole milk

This recipe provides all the sweetness of classic blueberry muffins, but with an immune-boosting and cancer-healing bonus. The blueberries, cinnamon, and nutmeg are all great sources of antioxidants and anticancer phytonutrients, while the flaxseed helps support hormonal balance and digestive health. It's best to buy the flaxseeds whole and grind them in a coffee grinder right before using them. You can also buy flax meal—just make sure to keep it refrigerated to prevent oxidation. To make this recipe dairy-free, substitute the milk with unsweetened coconut or almond milk.

1. Preheat the oven to 350°F. Lightly grease a 12-cup muffin tin.

2. In a large bowl, mix the flour, flaxseed, brown sugar, baking powder, cinnamon, nutmeg, and salt. Add the blueberries and toss to coat.

3. In a medium bowl, lightly beat the eggs with the milk.

4. Add the egg mixture to the flour mixture, stirring until just combined. Be careful not to overmix.

5. Pour the batter into the muffin tin, filling each cup two-thirds of the way. Bake for 30 minutes, or until a toothpick inserted into the center of a muffin comes out mostly clean.

6. Let the muffins cool in the pan for a few minutes, then transfer to a wire rack to cool completely. The muffins will keep in an airtight container at room temperature for up to 2 days, in the refrigerator for 1 week, or in the freezer for up to 3 months.

VARIATION TIP: If you'd like to increase the protein, add ⅔ cup chopped nuts, such as almonds, walnuts, or pecans, to the dry ingredients in step 2.

PER SERVING (1 MUFFIN): Calories: 194; Total fat: 7g; Sodium: 105mg; Carbohydrates: 31g; Fiber: 4g; Protein: 6g

# Sweet Potato Porridge

SERVES: 2 | PREP TIME: 10 Minutes | COOK TIME: 15 Minutes

SYMPTOMS: Nausea / Trouble Swallowing / Taste Changes / Sore Mouth or Throat / Unintentional Weight Loss

2 large sweet potatoes, peeled and cut into 1- to 2-inch cubes

1 cup unsweetened coconut milk

1 teaspoon ground cinnamon

Pinch sea salt

Raw almond butter, unsweetened shredded coconut, or fresh berries, for topping (optional)

I discovered this recipe when I decided to stop eating grains for a while. I really wanted a replacement for hot cereal in the morning, and so this recipe was born. It's sweet enough to pass as a morning treat, but there is no added sugar, and it provides a great dose of fiber. Much as with carrots, sweet potatoes are a superb source of antioxidants and anti-inflammatory nutrients. To add more calories, you can use canned full-fat coconut milk, melt in 1 to 2 tablespoons of coconut oil, stir in some nut or seed butter, or top with chopped nuts.

1. In a large pot, cover the sweet potatoes with water and bring to a boil over medium-high heat. Reduce the heat to low and simmer until the potatoes are soft enough to pierce easily with a fork, about 15 minutes. Drain.

2. Place the cooked sweet potatoes, coconut milk, cinnamon, and salt in a high-speed blender and mix on high power until smooth and creamy, 1 to 2 minutes. You can use more or less coconut milk depending on the texture you prefer. (Alternatively, use an immersion blender or potato masher to blend the potatoes in the pot.)

3. Divide the mixture between 2 bowls and enjoy as is, or top with any of your other favorite toppings. Store leftovers in an airtight container in the refrigerator for 3 to 5 days.

FLAVOR TIP: To enhance the flavor, sprinkle in vanilla extract or your favorite spice—such as ground cardamom, nutmeg, or pumpkin pie spice—or consider adding the grated zest and juice of one orange, plus a squeeze of lemon. The addition of citrus is especially nice if you're experiencing taste changes and don't have mouth sores.

PER SERVING: Calories: 135; Total fat: 2g; Sodium: 132mg; Carbohydrates: 27g; Fiber: 5g; Protein: 2g

# Veggie Breakfast Burritos

| MAKES: 4 | PREP TIME: 10 Minutes | COOK TIME: 20 Minutes |

SYMPTOMS: Fatigue / Anemia / Taste Changes / Unintentional Weight Loss / Diarrhea / Constipation

Hearty and full of flavor, breakfast burritos are a nice go-to meal to keep in your fridge or freezer. The bold flavors of garlic, onion, spices, and salsa are helpful when the taste buds become dull, while the protein, iron, and B vitamins in the eggs and black beans can counteract anemia and fatigue. If you want to add animal protein, you can use the Sausage and Roasted Veggie Hash (page 44) in place of the veggie filling. If you want to make it vegan, omit the cheese and substitute the eggs with the tofu variation of Turmeric Scrambled Eggs (page 38). If you want to store these burritos in the freezer (see Tip), just omit the avocado and salsa, which don't freeze well.

1 tablespoon plus 1 teaspoon extra-virgin olive oil or avocado oil, divided

3 garlic cloves, minced or pressed

1 medium onion, diced

1 medium sweet potato, cut into ½-inch cubes

1 red bell pepper, cored, seeded, and diced

1 green bell pepper, cored, seeded, and diced

1 teaspoon ground cumin

½ teaspoon chili powder

½ teaspoon sea salt, divided

¼ teaspoon freshly ground black pepper, divided

1 cup roughly chopped fresh kale

8 large eggs

2 tablespoons water

4 (12-inch) whole wheat or gluten-free tortillas

1 cup canned black beans, rinsed and drained

½ cup shredded sharp cheddar cheese

1 avocado, pitted, peeled, and sliced

Fresh Salsa (page 175) (optional)

Hot sauce of choice (optional)

1. Heat 1 tablespoon of the olive oil in a large skillet over medium heat. Add the garlic, onion, sweet potato, bell peppers, cumin, chili powder, ¼ teaspoon salt, and ⅛ teaspoon pepper. Stir to coat the veggies with the spices, then cover and cook for about 10 minutes, stirring occasionally, until the sweet potato is fork-tender. Add the kale and cook until wilted, about 2 minutes. Transfer the vegetable mixture to a plate.

2. In a medium bowl, whisk together the eggs, water, remaining ¼ teaspoon of salt, and remaining ⅛ teaspoon of pepper.

3. In the same skillet, heat the remaining 1 teaspoon of olive oil over medium heat. Pour in the egg mixture. When it starts to set around the edges, about 1 minute, use a heatproof spatula to push the cooked edges toward the center of the pan. Continue this action until the eggs are gathered in the center of the pan in fluffy curds. (This should take less than 5 minutes.) Break up the eggs with the spatula to make sure they are evenly cooked, then turn off the heat. The eggs should be moist but not runny.

4. To assemble the burritos, divide the eggs and vegetable mixture evenly among the tortillas. Top each with some of the black beans, cheese, and avocado. Add the salsa and hot sauce, if using. Fold the ends of the tortillas over the filling and snugly roll the burritos, ending seam side down. Serve warm. Store leftovers wrapped in parchment or foil in the refrigerator for up to 4 days.

PREP AHEAD TIP: To freeze, wrap each burrito individually in parchment paper or foil and place in a freezer-safe bag. Squeeze out all the air and seal. Freeze for up to 1 month. To reheat from frozen, unwrap the burrito, then rewrap in a damp paper towel. Microwave for 2 to 3 minutes, until warmed through.

PER SERVING (1 BURRITO): Calories: 577; Total fat: 31g; Sodium: 711mg; Carbohydrates: 49g; Fiber: 15g; Protein: 27g

# Turmeric Scrambled Eggs

| SERVES: 2 | PREP TIME: 5 Minutes | COOK TIME: 5 Minutes |

SYMPTOMS: Nausea / Fatigue / Trouble Swallowing / Anemia / Sore Mouth or Throat / Unintentional Weight Loss

4 large eggs

2 tablespoons water

½ teaspoon ground turmeric

¼ teaspoon sea salt

⅛ teaspoon freshly ground black pepper

1 teaspoon extra-virgin olive or avocado oil

Sliced avocado (optional)

Whole-grain or gluten-free bread, toasted (optional)

A plate of scrambled eggs is one of the fastest and easiest meals you can make that is also a good source of calories, protein, and healthy fat. Turmeric is such an important anticancer, anti-inflammatory spice, and it blends beautifully with eggs. You can start with less than the ½ teaspoon that the recipe calls for if you're unfamiliar with this spice, and if you love it, add more. It's also important to add a bit of black pepper in order to increase your body's absorption of the turmeric.

1. In a bowl, whisk together the eggs, water, turmeric, salt, and pepper until well blended, about 1 minute.

2. Heat the oil in a medium skillet over medium heat, until it shimmers. Pour in the egg mixture. When it starts to set around the edges, use a heatproof spatula to push the cooked edges toward the center of the pan. Continue this action until the eggs are gathered in the center of the pan in fluffy curds. Break up the eggs with the spatula to make sure they are evenly cooked, then turn off the heat. The eggs should be moist but not runny.

**3.** Serve immediately, topped with avocado slices, or with a slice of toast, if desired. Store leftovers in an airtight container in the refrigerator for 4 days.

VARIATION TIP: For a vegan option, substitute tofu for the eggs. Wrap an 8-ounce block of firm or extra-firm tofu in a towel, place it in a dish, and put a heavy object on top, such as a can of tomatoes, to press out the water. Let it sit for 5 minutes. Crumble the tofu with a fork into fine pieces. Heat the oil in a large skillet over medium heat, add the tofu, turmeric, salt, and pepper, and cook, stirring, until all the liquid is gone and the tofu is completely yellow and hot, about 5 minutes.

PER SERVING: Calories: 148; Total fat: 11g; Sodium: 358mg; Carbohydrates: 1g; Fiber: 0g; Protein: 11g

# Veggie Omelet

SERVES: 2 | PREP TIME: 5 Minutes | COOK TIME: 10 Minutes

SYMPTOMS: Fatigue / Trouble Swallowing / Anemia / Unintentional Weight Loss

5 large eggs

¼ teaspoon sea salt

⅛ teaspoon freshly ground black pepper

1 tablespoon extra-virgin olive oil

½ cup shredded cheese (such as cheddar, Emmentaler, or Gruyère)

1 avocado, pitted, peeled, and sliced

1 ripe medium tomato, sliced

4 fresh mushrooms (such as cremini, button, or shiitake), thinly sliced

1 cup chopped fresh spinach

2 tablespoons water

The eggs and spinach in this omelet are good sources of iron, while the tomatoes have vitamin C, which helps you absorb the iron better (though you might consider omitting these if you have mouth sores). The avocado adds extra calories and healthy fat. I like to use cheddar, Emmentaler, or Gruyère in this recipe, but you can use any cheese you like, or omit it altogether if you're dairy-free.

1. In a medium bowl, whisk together the eggs, salt, and pepper.

2. Heat a large skillet over medium-low heat. Drizzle a drop of water onto the surface to check the heat. When the water beads and moves around, add the olive oil, pour in the eggs, and let them spread over the bottom of the skillet. After 20 to 30 seconds, sprinkle the cheese evenly over the eggs.

3. Once the eggs have begun to set (the bottom should be firm but the top will still look a little wet) and the cheese is melted, add the avocado, tomato, mushrooms, and spinach over half of the omelet.

4. Carefully fold over the side of the omelet without the vegetables. You might need to use 2 spatulas to prevent the omelet from breaking. Using a spatula, move the omelet to the center of the pan, pour the water into the pan, cover, and cook until the omelet puffs up, about 5 minutes.

5. Remove from the heat. Divide the omelet in half with the spatula and serve immediately. Store leftovers in an airtight container in the refrigerator for 3 days.

PER SERVING: Calories: 537; Total fat: 42g; Sodium: 591mg; Carbohydrates: 17g; Fiber: 10g; Protein: 26g

# Egg and Veggie Sandwich

**SERVES: 2 to 4**  |  **PREP TIME: 5 Minutes**  |  **COOK TIME: 8 Minutes**

**SYMPTOMS:** Nausea / Fatigue / Anemia / Unintentional Weight Loss

2 tablespoons unsalted butter (preferably grass-fed), ghee, or coconut oil, divided

4 large eggs

Pinch sea salt

4 slices whole-grain or gluten-free bread, toasted

Ground turmeric

1 avocado, pitted, peeled, and sliced

1 cup chopped fresh spinach

Freshly ground black pepper

An egg and veggie sandwich is my go-to meal when I don't know what to make for lunch. It provides a balanced mix of protein, fiber, and healthy fat, and it incorporates turmeric into your diet.

1. Heat a large skillet over medium heat. Drizzle a drop of water onto the surface. When the water beads and moves around, add 1 tablespoon of the butter. As soon as it melts, crack the eggs, one at a time, into the pan, leaving a bit of room between them.

2. Reduce the heat to medium-low and cook until the egg whites are mostly solidified, 3 to 5 minutes. Season with salt. Flip the eggs, then turn off the heat.

3. Spread the remaining 1 tablespoon of butter on the toast slices. Sprinkle each with turmeric as desired. Divide the avocado slices and spinach among them.

4. Top each toast with an egg and some pepper. Serve immediately.

**VARIATION TIPS:** In place of spinach, consider arugula, baby kale, or any tender leafy greens. Instead of using them raw, try sautéing them first in a bit of butter or oil.

PER SERVING: Calories: 568; Total fat: 38g; Sodium: 434mg; Carbohydrates: 36g; Fiber: 13g; Protein: 23g

# Spinach and Black Bean Breakfast Bowl

30

VG

| SERVES: 2 | PREP TIME: 10 Minutes | COOK TIME: 10 Minutes |
| --- | --- | --- |

SYMPTOMS: Fatigue / Anemia / Taste Changes / Constipation

Here's a savory breakfast that provides a powerful dose of vitamins and nutrients. The spinach, black beans, and quinoa are all rich in iron, while the vitamin C in the tomatoes helps with the absorption of that iron. The beans and quinoa provide digestive-supporting fiber, and the eggs and beans are packed with healthy protein.

2 large eggs

1 tablespoon extra-virgin olive oil

10 cherry tomatoes, halved

1 cup chopped fresh spinach

1 cup cooked quinoa

1 cup canned black beans, rinsed and drained

Sea salt

Freshly ground black pepper

1 avocado, pitted, peeled, and sliced

1.  Bring a large pot of water to a boil over medium-high heat. Reduce the heat to low.

2.  Crack each egg into a separate ramekin, small bowl, or cup. When the water is simmering, gently slip the eggs into the water one at a time. Turn off the heat, cover the pot, and poach until the whites are cooked through but the yolks are still runny, about 4 minutes. Remove the eggs with a slotted spoon and transfer to a paper towel–lined plate.

3.  Heat the olive oil in a large skillet over medium heat. Add the tomatoes and cook until blistered, 3 to 4 minutes. Add the spinach and cook until just wilted, about 1 minute. Stir in the quinoa and beans and cook to warm through. Remove from the heat and season with salt and pepper.

4.  Divide the tomato mixture between 2 bowls, top each with half the avocado slices and an egg, and serve immediately.

PER SERVING: Calories: 567; Total fat: 29g; Sodium: 253mg; Carbohydrates: 60g; Fiber: 22g; Protein: 25g

# Sausage and Roasted Veggie Hash

| SERVES: 4 | PREP TIME: 10 Minutes | COOK TIME: 20 Minutes |
| --- | --- | --- |

**SYMPTOMS:** Fatigue / Anemia / Taste Changes / Unintentional Weight Loss

8 ounces baby Yukon
Gold or red or purple
potatoes, quartered

1 small sweet potato, cut into
bite-size pieces

2 cups Brussels sprouts,
halved or quartered

2 tablespoons extra-virgin
olive oil, divided

Sea salt

Freshly ground black pepper

1 small onion, diced

1 red bell pepper, cored,
seeded, and diced

3 or 4 links cooked nitrate-free
chicken or turkey sausage,
cut into bite-size pieces

3 garlic cloves, minced
or pressed

1 tablespoon herbes
de Provence

2 cups roughly chopped
fresh spinach

A breakfast dish that's both strengthening and satisfying, this hash provides protein, fiber, and many cancer-healing phytonutrients. It's a great way to get your vegetables in the morning, including cancer-fighting cruciferous Brussels sprouts. I enjoy this hash on its own, but it's also delicious topped with a runny egg.

1. Preheat the oven to 400°F. Line a baking sheet with parchment paper.

2. Put the potatoes, sweet potato, and Brussels sprouts on the baking sheet. Drizzle with 1 tablespoon of the oil, season with a pinch each of salt and pepper, and toss to coat well. Spread out in a single layer. Roast until tender and golden brown, about 20 minutes, stirring halfway through to ensure even cooking.

3.  While the vegetables are roasting, heat the remaining 1 tablespoon of oil in a large skillet over medium heat. Add the onion and cook, stirring occasionally, until translucent, about 3 minutes. Add the bell pepper, sausage, garlic, and herbes de Provence and stir to combine. Cook, stirring frequently, until the peppers are soft and the sausage is heated through, 8 to 10 minutes. Add the spinach, cover, and cook for a few minutes more, until wilted. Remove from the heat.

4.  Stir the roasted vegetables into the sausage mixture.

5.  Serve warm. Store leftovers in an airtight container in the refrigerator for up to 4 days or in the freezer for up to 1 month.

PER SERVING: Calories: 294; Total fat: 14g; Sodium: 519mg; Carbohydrates: 24g; Fiber: 5g; Protein: 19g

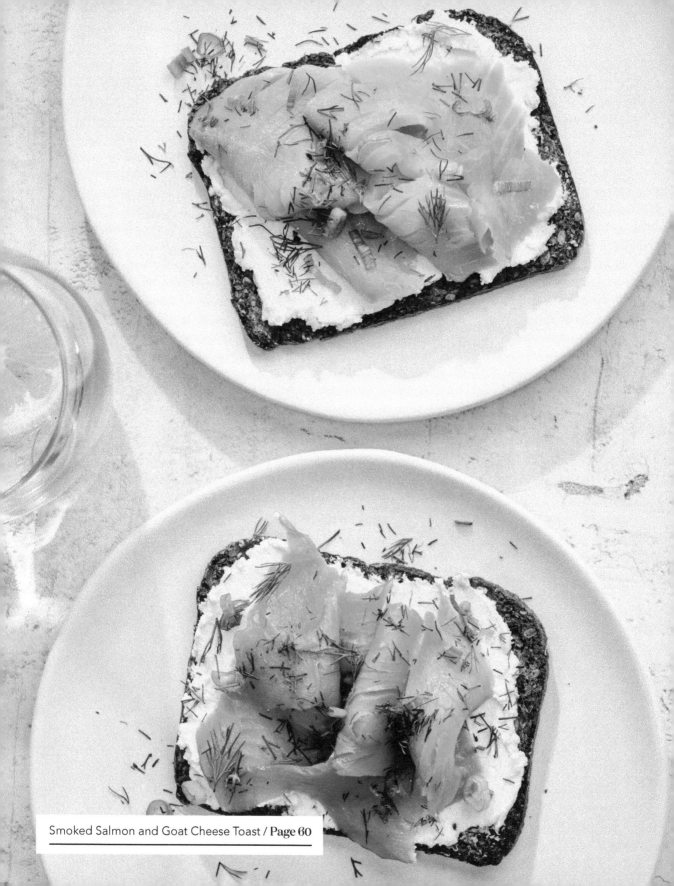

Smoked Salmon and Goat Cheese Toast / **Page 60**

# CHAPTER 3

# Protein-Packed Snacks

# Cinnamon-Spiced Apple Compote with Nut Butter

| SERVES: 2 to 4 | PREP TIME: 5 Minutes | COOK TIME: 20 Minutes |
|---|---|---|

SYMPTOMS: Nausea / Fatigue / Trouble Swallowing / Sore Mouth or Throat / Diarrhea / Constipation

This compote is by far one of my favorite quick-and-easy sweet snacks. Apples are an excellent source of fiber and can aid both constipation and diarrhea. Cooking them down makes it much easier to chew and swallow the fruit, if you're having any difficulty with that. The spices support digestion in addition to being immune supporting and a good source of cancer-healing phytonutrients. This recipe doubles well, and is a great topping for yogurt, hot cereal, or even Vegan Banana-Walnut Ice Cream (page 50).

| | | |
|---|---|---|
| Apple, cored and chopped into bite-size pieces | 1 teaspoon ground cinnamon | ½ teaspoon sea salt |
| ½ teaspoon grated fresh ginger, or ¼ teaspoon ground ginger | ½ teaspoon ground cardamom | ⅓ cup water |
| | 2 to 4 whole cloves | 4 tablespoons raw almond butter or nut butter of your choice |

1. Combine the apples, ginger, cinnamon, cardamom, cloves, salt, and water in a small saucepan, stir together, and cook, covered, over medium-low heat until simmering, about 5 minutes.

2. Remove the lid and continue to cook until the apples are tender enough to pierce easily with a fork, about 15 minutes. If the water evaporates during cooking, add more as needed.

3. To serve, spoon the warm apples into bowls and drizzle with 1 to 2 tablespoons of the almond butter. Store in an airtight container in the refrigerator for up to 1 week.

PER SERVING: Calories: 217; Total fat: 9g; Sodium: 236mg; Carbohydrates: 35g; Fiber: 7g; Protein: 4g

# Dark Chocolate Brownie Bites

**MAKES:** 8 to 10 Balls | **PREP TIME:** 5 Minutes | ///////////////

**SYMPTOMS:** Fatigue / Anemia / Unintentional Weight Loss / Constipation

1 cup pitted dates

½ cup raw walnuts

⅓ cup raw cacao powder or unsweetened Dutch-process cocoa powder

1 teaspoon vanilla extract

¼ teaspoon sea salt

With these low-sugar, vegan, flourless treats, you can enjoy all the yummy gooeyness of fudgy brownies without the inflammatory ingredients. These brownie bites don't require turning on an oven and are simple enough for your kids to make. In addition to satisfying cravings, dark chocolate and dates are excellent sources of iron and other important minerals.

1. In a high-speed blender or a food processor, process the dates, walnuts, cacao, vanilla, and salt until combined and sticking together, about 1 minute.

2. Roll the mixture into balls about 1 inch in diameter. Eat immediately, or store in an airtight container in the refrigerator for up to 1 week.

PER SERVING (1 BALL): Calories: 109; Total fat: 5g; Sodium: 59mg; Carbohydrates: 17g; Fiber: 3g; Protein: 2g

# Vegan Banana-Walnut Ice Cream

| SERVES: 2 | PREP TIME: 10 Minutes | FREEZER TIME: 1 Hour |

**SYMPTOMS:** Nausea / Fatigue / Trouble Swallowing / Taste Changes / Sore Mouth or Throat / Diarrhea

3 large ripe bananas, peeled and sliced into coins

2 tablespoons chopped raw walnuts or other mix-ins (see Tip)

**VARIATION TIP:** The pairing potential for bananas is practically infinite. Some of my favorite mix-ins are dark chocolate chips and walnuts; cocoa powder and peanut or almond butter; coconut milk and shredded coconut; frozen berries and vanilla extract; ground cinnamon or cardamom and ginger.

Simple yet satisfying, this creamy frozen treat is perfect when you're dealing with nausea, a sore mouth, or taste changes. It has no added sugar and can easily be adjusted to boost calories or protein, or change the flavor profile. It doesn't require an ice cream maker and is super quick to throw together when you're craving something sweet. Keep bananas in the freezer so you can make this at a moment's notice.

1. Freeze the banana slices on a parchment-lined baking sheet for at least 1 hour, until the slices are frozen solid.

2. In a food processor or high-speed blender, process the bananas until smooth, about 4 minutes. The mixture will transform from crumbly to gooey to creamy. When it's finished, it should look like soft-serve ice cream.

3. Stir in the walnuts and enjoy immediately or return to the freezer in an airtight container to let it solidify.

PER SERVING: Calories: 229; Total fat: 5g; Sodium: 2mg; Carbohydrates: 47g; Fiber: 6g; Protein: 3g

# Healthy Trail Mix

MAKES: **4½ Cups** | PREP TIME: **10 Minutes**

**SYMPTOMS:** Fatigue / Taste Changes / Unintentional Weight Loss / Diarrhea / Constipation

½ cup raw almonds

½ cup raw walnuts

½ cup raw pecans

½ cup raw Brazil nuts

½ cup raw pumpkin seeds

½ cup unsweetened dried cherries

½ cup raisins

½ cup chopped dark chocolate or chocolate chips

½ cup unsweetened shredded coconut

¼ teaspoon sea salt

**VARIATION TIP:** To make your own mix, combine 1½ cups of your favorite nuts, 1 cup dried fruit, 1 cup seeds, and ½ cup other mix-ins, such as dark chocolate chunks, shredded coconut, or chopped crystallized ginger. A pinch of seasoning, such as sea salt, ground cinnamon, nutmeg, ginger, or curry powder, can go a long way. Consider toasting your nuts and seeds in the oven at 350°F for added flavor.

During cancer treatment and recovery, it's important to not skip meals, especially when you're trying to maintain your weight, energy, and strength. Which is why trail mix is great to have on hand. It's a quick and easy snack, especially when you're on the go. When you're out at doctors' appointments all day and you don't know when the next meal is coming, pack some trail mix, grab a piece of fruit and a bottle of water, and you're covered. Whenever possible, choose raw nuts and seeds, so you can benefit from their oils and antioxidant content, and to minimize the intake of added salt. And when buying dried fruit, go for the unsweetened, unsulfured varieties, as sulfites can cause inflammatory reactions.

Combine all the ingredients in a large bowl and mix well. The mix will stay fresh in an airtight container at room temperature for 1 month.

PER SERVING (½ CUP): Calories: 326; Total fat: 27g; Sodium: 64mg; Carbohydrates: 18g; Fiber: 5g; Protein: 8g

# Carrot, Apple, and Walnut Muffins

**MAKES:** 18 Muffins | **PREP TIME:** 10 Minutes | **COOK TIME:** 20 Minutes

**SYMPTOMS:** Nausea / Trouble Swallowing / Sore Mouth or Throat / Unintentional Weight Loss / Diarrhea / Constipation

1¾ cups whole wheat or
   gluten-free flour
1 teaspoon baking soda
¼ teaspoon sea salt
2 teaspoons ground cinnamon
¾ cup honey or maple syrup
½ cup coconut oil, melted
½ cup unsweetened
   applesauce
2 teaspoons vanilla extract
3 large eggs
1¼ cups shredded apple
   (1 large apple)
1¼ cups shredded carrots
   (2 large carrots)
1 cup chopped walnuts
½ cup unsweetened
   shredded coconut

These muffins are easy to make and are loaded with healthy anticancer nutrients, fiber, and healthy fat. They also provide some protein, although you can add more by serving them with a spoonful of nut or seed butter. As with all muffins, the trick is to make sure you don't overmix the batter, which leads to a denser, tougher muffin.

1. Preheat the oven to 375°F. Lightly grease a 12-cup and a 6-cup muffin tin. (If you don't have 2 muffin tins, bake in 2 batches, washing the tin and greasing it again.)

2. In a medium bowl, whisk together the flour, baking soda, salt, and cinnamon.

3. In a large bowl, whisk together the honey, coconut oil, applesauce, vanilla, and eggs until well blended. Stir in the apple and carrots.

4. Stir in the dry ingredients, making sure not to overmix. Fold in the walnuts and coconut.

5.  Pour the batter into the muffin tins, filling each two-thirds of the way. Bake for about 18 minutes, until a toothpick inserted in the center comes out mostly clean.

6.  Let the muffins cool in the pans for a few minutes, then transfer to a wire rack to cool completely. Store the muffins in an airtight container or resealable storage bag at room temperature for up to 2 days, in the refrigerator for 1 week, or in the freezer for up to 3 months.

PER SERVING (1 MUFFIN): Calories: 200; Total fat: 12g; Sodium: 116mg; Carbohydrates: 21g; Fiber: 3g; Protein: 4g

# Curry Hummus

**MAKES:** About 1½ Cups  |  **PREP TIME:** 10 Minutes

**SYMPTOMS:** Nausea / Fatigue / Anemia / Trouble Swallowing / Taste Changes / Unintentional Weight Loss / Diarrhea

¼ cup raw tahini

2 tablespoons extra-virgin olive oil

1½ cups cooked chickpeas, or 1 (15-ounce) can chickpeas, rinsed and drained

2 tablespoons cold water, or more as needed

¼ cup freshly squeezed lemon juice (from 1 large lemon), or more as desired

1 garlic clove, roughly chopped

1 teaspoon curry powder

1 teaspoon ground ginger

½ teaspoon sea salt, or more as needed

Raw or cooked vegetables, apple slices, or whole-grain crackers

**MAKE IT EASIER TIP:**
If you don't have the time or energy to make hummus, doctor a 16-ounce container of store-bought hummus by adding ginger, curry, and maybe some lemon juice.

Hummus is so easy to make from scratch, and is a great source of fiber, protein, healthy fat, iron, and calcium, thanks to the nutrient content of chickpeas, tahini, and olive oil. Adding the garlic, curry, and ginger gives it a great flavor kick, but also a healthy dose of anti-inflammatory, anticancer phytonutrients. Try this hummus on Avocado Hummus Toast (page 59).

1.  Pulse the tahini and olive oil in a food processor until blended. Add the chickpeas, water, lemon juice, garlic, curry powder, ginger, and salt and process until the hummus is smooth and creamy, about 5 minutes, or until you've reached your desired consistency. The longer you process, the smoother it will be. Add more water if needed for a smoother, lighter consistency. Season with more salt and lemon juice, if desired.

2.  Serve with raw or cooked vegetables, sliced apples, or whole-grain crackers. Store leftovers in an airtight container in the refrigerator for up to 1 week.

PER SERVING (¼ CUP): Calories: 172; Total fat: 11g; Sodium: 170mg; Carbohydrates: 15g; Fiber: 4g; Protein: 5g

# Green Pea Guacamole

SERVES: 6 | PREP TIME: 10 Minutes

SYMPTOMS: Fatigue / Taste Changes / Unintentional Weight Loss

Many of the health benefits of guacamole are thanks to the avocados, which are loaded with healthy fats while also being good sources of fiber, vitamin E, B vitamins, potassium, and magnesium. I like the addition of peas or edamame, which provides protein without changing the color or the flavor. When you're trying to make every bite count and get in as much protein as possible, this is an easy way to accomplish that. To keep the guacamole from turning brown, press a piece of plastic wrap directly onto the surface before refrigerating. Give it a good stir before serving. This guacamole makes a great dip, but you can also use it as a sandwich spread or a topping for tacos, chicken, or even fish.

1 cup frozen peas or edamame, thawed

1 medium jalapeño pepper (for less spice, discard seeds)

½ cup chopped red or white onion (1 small onion)

1 garlic clove

2 tablespoons coarsely chopped fresh cilantro leaves

3 medium avocados, pitted, peeled, and diced

Grated zest and juice of 1 lime, or more as desired

1 teaspoon sea salt, or more as desired

½ teaspoon freshly ground black pepper

½ cup diced ripe tomato (optional)

Raw or cooked vegetables, tortilla chips, or whole-grain crackers

1. In a food processor, process the peas, jalapeño, onion, garlic, and cilantro until a slightly chunky paste forms.

2. In a medium bowl, combine the diced avocado, lime zest and juice, salt, pepper, and pea mixture. Mash until well combined but still a little chunky. Stir in the diced tomato, if using. Taste and add more salt and lime juice, if desired.

3. Serve immediately with raw or cooked vegetables, tortilla chips, or whole-grain crackers. Store in an airtight container in the refrigerator for 2 to 3 days.

PER SERVING: Calories: 223; Total fat: 17g; Sodium: 316mg; Carbohydrates: 17g; Fiber: 10g; Protein: 6g

# Lemon and Rosemary Bean Dip

**MAKES:** About 1½ Cups | **PREP TIME:** 10 Minutes | ///////////////////////

**SYMPTOMS:** Nausea / Fatigue / Trouble Swallowing / Anemia Taste Changes / Unintentional Weight Loss / Diarrhea

1 (15-ounce) can white beans, rinsed and drained

1 to 3 garlic cloves, peeled

½ teaspoon sea salt, or more as desired

Juice of 1 large lemon (about 2 tablespoons)

¼ cup extra-virgin olive oil

1 tablespoon minced fresh rosemary, or 1 teaspoon dried

Grated zest of 2 lemons

Raw or cooked vegetables, sliced apples, whole-grain crackers, or chips (preferably fried in avocado oil or coconut oil)

White beans, such as cannellini, are a great source of fiber and protein. The olive oil in this easy dip provides healthy fat, while the lemon zest, rosemary, and garlic offer a number of anticancer, anti-inflammatory, and antibacterial phytonutrients. Besides adding some healthy kick to your snacks, dips are an excellent way to help you eat more vegetables. Try an assortment, such as jicama, carrots, cucumber, cherry tomatoes, celery, radish, bell pepper, green beans, broccoli, and cauliflower, with all the dips in this chapter.

1. In a food processor, process the beans, garlic, salt, and lemon juice while adding the oil in a steady stream. Process until smooth and creamy.

2. Transfer the dip to a serving bowl. Stir in the rosemary and lemon zest, and add more salt, if desired.

3. Serve with raw or cooked vegetables, apples, whole-grain crackers, or chips, or use as a sandwich spread. Store in an airtight container in the refrigerator for up to 1 week.

PER SERVING (¼ CUP): Calories: 148; Total fat: 9g; Sodium: 158mg; Carbohydrates: 13g; Fiber: 3g; Protein: 4g

# Miso-Tahini Dip

**MAKES: About ¾ Cup** | **PREP TIME: 5 Minutes**

**SYMPTOMS:** Fatigue / Anemia / Taste Changes / Constipation

½ cup raw tahini

1½ tablespoons red miso

¼ cup water

2 garlic cloves, minced
  or pressed

Raw or cooked vegetables,
  sliced apples, whole-grain
  crackers, or chips

Miso, a fermented soybean paste, adds a rich burst of umami to food in addition to healthy probiotics, which are great for digestive support. Miso and tahini are good sources of protein, and both are helpful at supporting hormonal balance, thanks to the phytoestrogen content in soybeans and sesame seeds. Make sure you choose an organic traditional miso without any additives. This dip is also great as a spread for toast, sandwiches, or wraps.

1. In a medium bowl, stir together the tahini and miso until well combined. Add the water gradually while stirring. The mixture will first thicken, then turn smooth and creamy. Stop adding the water once you've reached this consistency. Add the garlic and mix well.

2. Serve with raw or cooked vegetables, apples, whole-grain crackers, or chips. Store in an airtight container in the refrigerator for up to 1 week.

PER SERVING (¼ CUP): Calories: 258; Total fat: 22g; Sodium: 363mg; Carbohydrates: 11g; Fiber: 4g; Protein: 8g

# Garlic-Herb Yogurt Dip

**(5)**
**(30)**
**VG**

| MAKES: **About 1½ Cups** | PREP TIME: **10 Minutes** | //////////// |

1 cup plain full-fat
  Greek yogurt
2 tablespoons chopped
  fresh chives
1 garlic clove, minced
  or pressed
2 tablespoons freshly
  squeezed lemon juice
2 tablespoons chopped
  fresh dill
½ teaspoon sea salt
¼ teaspoon freshly ground
  black pepper
Raw or cooked vegetables,
  sliced apples, whole-grain
  crackers, or pita chips

Whole-fat Greek-style yogurt is your best choice for maximizing the calorie and protein content of this recipe. Adding fresh herbs, garlic, and lemon juice enhances the flavor and adds anticancer, anti-inflammatory phytonutrients. Garlic is also a great detox supporter, and the fiber in garlic promotes the growth of healthy bacteria in the digestive tract. Combined with the healthy bacteria found in yogurt, this dip will support good digestion and healthy immunity. It is great as a sandwich spread, or pair it with grilled lamb, chicken, or fish.

1. In a medium bowl, stir together the yogurt, chives, garlic, lemon juice, and dill. Season with the salt and pepper.

2. Serve with raw or cooked vegetables, apples, whole-grain crackers, or pita chips. Store in an air-tight container in the refrigerator for up to 1 week (the garlic flavor will become more pronounced the longer it sits).

VARIATION TIPS: To make this dip more like tzatziki, omit the chives and use 1 peeled and seeded cucumber, chopped into ¼-inch pieces. To make it dairy-free, use a plant-based yogurt.

PER SERVING (¼ CUP): Calories: 34; Total fat: 2g; Sodium: 174mg; Carbohydrates: 4g; Fiber: 1g; Protein: 2g

# Avocado Hummus Toast

SERVES: 2 | PREP TIME: **5 Minutes**

**SYMPTOMS:** Nausea / Fatigue / Anemia / Taste Changes / Unintentional Weight Loss / Diarrhea

¼ cup hummus

2 slices whole-grain or gluten-free bread, toasted

1 avocado, pitted, peeled, and sliced

1 ripe medium tomato, sliced, or 6 cherry tomatoes, halved

Although this snack has only four simple ingredients, it's loaded with fiber, protein, and healthy fat. The hummus is a good source of iron, which can help with anemia, while the tomato provides vitamin C to help you absorb the iron better. You may want to omit the tomato if you have mouth sores. To help boost calories, add a drizzle of olive oil to the toast before adding the hummus. This recipe is delicious with either store-bought or homemade hummus, like the Curry Hummus (page 54).

Spread half the hummus on each piece of toast. Top with the avocado and tomato slices, divided evenly. Serve.

PER SERVING: Calories: 317; Total fat: 19g; Sodium: 180mg; Carbohydrates: 32g; Fiber: 12g; Protein: 9g

5

30

# Smoked Salmon and Goat Cheese Toast

SERVES: **2**  |  PREP TIME: **5 Minutes**  |

SYMPTOMS: Fatigue / Anemia / Taste Changes / Unintentional Weight Loss

3 ounces (about ¼ cup) goat cheese (chèvre)

2 slices whole-grain or gluten-free bread, toasted

3 ounces (about 3 pieces) thinly sliced smoked salmon

2 teaspoons thinly sliced scallion whites

2 tablespoons chopped fresh dill

Salmon is rich in omega-3 fats, which help lower inflammation and support the immune system. Fish contains vitamin D, and is one of only a few foods that does. Despite all these health benefits, smoked fish does contain a lot of salt, so be mindful to minimize salt elsewhere. For extra calories, smear on a little butter or ghee before adding the goat cheese.

Spread half the goat cheese on each piece of toast. Top with the salmon, scallion, and dill. Serve.

VARIATION TIP: Instead of goat cheese, try cream cheese, crème fraîche, or Garlic-Herb Yogurt Dip (page 58).

PER SERVING: Calories: 232; Total fat: 12g; Sodium: 555mg; Carbohydrates: 11g; Fiber: 2g; Protein: 19g

# Avocado Tuna Boats

SERVES: **2**  |  PREP TIME: **5 Minutes**

SYMPTOMS: Fatigue / Anemia / Unintentional Weight Loss / Constipation

1 (5-ounce) can wild-caught water-packed light tuna, drained

1 large avocado, halved, pitted, and chopped, hollowed-out skins reserved

1 ripe medium tomato, diced

1 celery stalk, chopped

Small handful fresh flat-leaf parsley, chopped

Juice of 1 lemon

½ teaspoon freshly ground black pepper

Raw or cooked vegetables, mixed greens, or toasted whole-grain bread (optional)

A good dietary goal is to eat 2 servings of wild-caught oily fish each week. It is a great source of protein and vital omega-3 fatty acids. Omega-3 fats help lower inflammation and support immunity, healing, and cancer recovery. For this recipe, I suggest choosing unsalted light tuna packed in water, as it's been found to be the lowest in mercury. This recipe also contains healthy fat and fiber from the avocado, as well as anticancer phytonutrients from the tomato, celery, and parsley.

1. In a small bowl, combine the tuna, avocado, tomato, celery, parsley, lemon juice, and pepper and mix with a fork, smashing the avocado.

2. Scoop the salad back into the avocado skins, or serve in 2 bowls with raw vegetables, over mixed greens, or on a slice of whole-grain or gluten-free toast. The salad is best eaten immediately.

FLAVOR BOOST TIP: For even more flavor, add chopped red onion or minced garlic; herbs such as fresh dill, thyme, or rosemary; or a touch of heat, like cayenne or diced jalapeño.

PER SERVING: Calories: 275; Total fat: 17g; Sodium: 46mg; Carbohydrates: 17g; Fiber: 10g; Protein: 18g

**30**

**VG**

# Spinach Egg Salad

| SERVES: 3 | PREP TIME: 10 Minutes | COOK TIME: 10 Minutes |
| --- | --- | --- |

SYMPTOMS: Fatigue / Anemia / Unintentional Weight Loss / Constipation

6 large eggs

1 (10-ounce) package frozen spinach, thawed

⅓ cup mayonnaise

3 tablespoons plain full-fat Greek yogurt

2 teaspoons Dijon mustard

¼ teaspoon sea salt

⅛ teaspoon freshly ground black pepper

Raw vegetables, whole-grain crackers, or mixed greens

This simple egg salad offers yet another way you can add leafy greens to your snacks or meals. Eggs are a great source of protein, healthy fat, iron, and immune-boosting nutrients like vitamin A, vitamin D, and selenium. Feel free to add herbs, like fresh dill or parsley, or vegetables, like chopped celery, minced scallions, or pickles, to bulk it up. Try making your own Healthy Homemade Mayonnaise (page 176), as store-bought mayonnaise often contains inflammatory oil, added sugar, and preservatives.

1. Place the eggs in a large saucepan, cover with water by 1 inch, cover the pan with a lid, and bring to a boil over high heat. Reduce the heat to medium-high and boil for 6 to 7 minutes. Drain and rinse the eggs in cold water, or transfer to a large bowl filled with ice water. Once cool, peel the eggs and roughly chop.

2. While the eggs are cooking, drain the spinach in a colander in the sink. Use a wooden spoon to press out as much liquid as possible.

3. In a medium bowl, combine the mayonnaise, yogurt, mustard, and salt. Add the spinach and chopped eggs. Mix well and season with pepper.

4. Divide evenly into 3 portions and serve with raw vegetables or whole-grain crackers, or on top of mixed greens. (It's also great in a sandwich.) Store in an airtight container for 3 to 5 days in the refrigerator.

VARIATION TIP: If you use a store-bought mayonnaise in this recipe, choose one that is made with olive or avocado oil, both of which are healthier anti-inflammatory fats.

PER SERVING: Calories: 338; Total fat: 29g; Sodium: 543mg; Carbohydrates: 5g; Fiber: 2g; Protein: 16g

# Lemon-Herb Chicken Salad

| SERVES: 4 | PREP TIME: 10 Minutes | COOK TIME: 35 Minutes |

SYMPTOMS: Fatigue / Anemia / Taste Changes / Sore Mouth or Throat /
Unintentional Weight Loss

3 or 4 boneless, skinless chicken breasts (about 1 pound)

½ teaspoon sea salt, or more as needed

¼ teaspoon freshly ground black pepper, or more as needed

½ to ¾ cup mayonnaise, store-bought or Healthy Homemade Mayonnaise (page 176)

1 teaspoon chopped fresh flat-leaf parsley

2 teaspoons chopped fresh chives

1 teaspoon chopped fresh dill, or ¼ teaspoon dried

1½ teaspoons chopped fresh oregano, or ½ teaspoon dried

1 tablespoon fresh lemon juice

Raw vegetables, whole-grain crackers, or mixed greens

Equally good with crackers or on its own in a bowl, chicken salad is a great protein-packed food to have in your fridge to fuel your recovery. The fresh herbs and lemon juice not only provide a bright flavor but also add antioxidants, antimicrobial benefits, and anticancer phytonutrients. To help with taste changes, you can vary the flavor and texture of this recipe by adding ¼ cup of chopped celery, 2 tablespoons of finely chopped red onion, ½ cup of seedless red grapes (halved), and/or ½ cup of chopped pecans, almonds, or walnuts.

1.  Preheat the oven to 400°F. Line a baking sheet with parchment paper.

2.  Arrange the chicken breasts on the sheet and sprinkle with the salt and pepper. Bake for 15 minutes, flip the breasts, and bake for 15 to 20 minutes longer, until the chicken is cooked through and the internal temperature is at least 165°F. Let the chicken cool, then chop into small pieces.

3. In a medium bowl, combine the mayonnaise with the parsley, chives, dill, oregano, and lemon juice. Add the chopped chicken and stir to coat. Add more mayonnaise, if desired. Season with salt and pepper, as desired.

4. Serve with raw vegetables or whole-grain crackers, or over mixed greens. (It's also great in a sandwich.) Store in an airtight container in the refrigerator for up to 4 days.

PER SERVING: Calories: 203; Total fat: 8g; Sodium: 315mg; Carbohydrates: 5g; Fiber: 0g; Protein: 26g

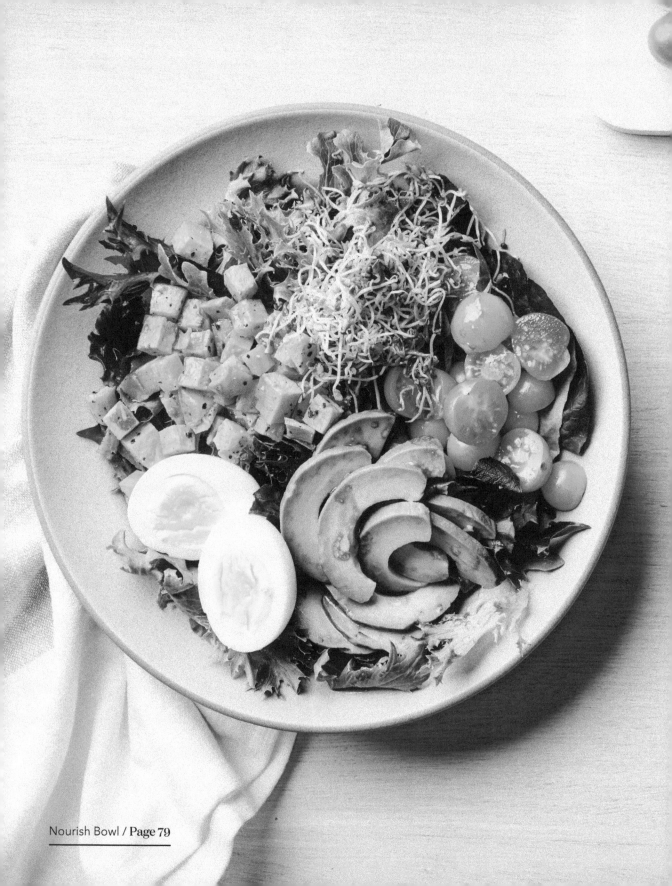

# CHAPTER 4

# Vegetables and Salads

# Roasted Sweet Potato Fries

| SERVES: 4 | PREP TIME: 15 Minutes | COOK TIME: 25 Minutes |

SYMPTOMS: Nausea / Taste Changes / Sore Mouth or Throat / Diarrhea / Constipation

3 large sweet potatoes,
  peeled and cut into
  long sticks
2 tablespoons extra-virgin
  olive or avocado oil
¼ teaspoon sea salt
1 teaspoon dried rosemary

VARIATION TIPS: I love my vegetables roasted with sea salt and rosemary, but you can use any herb or spice you like. Try dried oregano, dried thyme, herbes de Provence, ground cumin, curry powder, ground turmeric, or chili powder. You also can roast any vegetable you like, including some great anticancer veggies such as beets, carrots, tomatoes, garlic, broccoli, cauliflower, or Brussels sprouts, using the method in this recipe; the temperature will be the same but the cooking time may vary.

Roasting is one of my absolute favorite ways to prepare vegetables—it's easy and never disappoints. My kids actually prefer these sweet potato fries to the regular version. Sweet potatoes help maintain balanced blood sugar and are a great source of fiber, antioxidants, and anti-inflammatory nutrients. It's important to cut them all roughly the same size so they cook evenly.

1. Preheat the oven to 400°F. Line a baking sheet with parchment paper.

2. Arrange the sweet potatoes in a single layer on the baking sheet. Drizzle the oil over the sweet potatoes, sprinkle with the salt and rosemary, and toss to coat. I like to use my hands. Rearrange on the baking sheet in a single layer.

3. Roast, rotating the pan halfway through and turning the sweet potatoes once or twice, until the sweet potatoes are golden brown and tender, about 25 minutes.

4. Serve warm. Store leftovers in an airtight container in the refrigerator for up to 5 days.

PER SERVING: Calories: 146; Total fat: 7g; Sodium: 170mg; Carbohydrates: 20g; Fiber: 3g; Protein: 2g

# Golden Cauliflower

5
30
OP
V

| SERVES: 4 | PREP: 5 Minutes | COOK: 10 to 15 Minutes |
|---|---|---|

SYMPTOMS: Nausea / Fatigue / Anemia / Taste Changes / Constipation

2 tablespoons coconut oil

1 tablespoon ground turmeric
or curry powder

1 head cauliflower, cored and
cut into small florets

½ teaspoon sea salt

¼ teaspoon freshly ground
black pepper

Cauliflower is an important anticancer vegetable. As part of the cruciferous family, it supports detoxification, hormone balance, and immunity. It's also an excellent source of fiber, which aids healthy digestion. Turmeric is a spice that offers anticancer phytonutrients, antioxidants, and antimicrobial and anti-inflammatory benefits. The coconut oil provides healthy fat in addition to having antioxidants and antimicrobial benefits. This dish, with its powerhouse of benefits, is easy to make and so delicious.

1. Heat the oil and turmeric in a large skillet over medium-high heat. Add the cauliflower, salt, and pepper and toss to coat. Cook for about 5 minutes, until the cauliflower starts to brown. Reduce the heat to medium-low, add a few tablespoons of water, and cover. Simmer for another 5 to 10 minutes, until the cauliflower is tender.

2. Serve immediately as a side dish or as a topping for salad, or in a Nourish Bowl (page 79). Store leftovers in an airtight container in the refrigerator for 3 to 5 days.

PER SERVING: Calories: 80; Total fat: 7g; Sodium: 253mg; Carbohydrates: 4g; Fiber: 2g; Protein: 2g

# Easy Ratatouille

| SERVES: 4 | PREP: 10 Minutes | COOK: 30 to 40 Minutes |

SYMPTOMS: Anemia / Taste Changes / Constipation

1 large or 2 medium zucchini, cut into bite-size pieces

1 large onion, cut into bite-size pieces

1 small eggplant, cut into bite-size pieces

4 ripe large tomatoes, preferably heirloom, cut into bite-size pieces

4 large garlic cloves, minced or pressed

2 tablespoons extra-virgin olive oil

½ teaspoon sea salt

1 tablespoon herbes de Provence

This colorful, nutrient-rich dish has become a staple on our summer table. There are many different ways to make ratatouille. Baking in the oven is my favorite method, but you can also prepare it on the stovetop or on a grill. Sometimes we eat our ratatouille as the main dish by mixing in some white beans for protein and serving it with a side salad. Other times we use it as a side dish to accompany fish, chicken, or meat. Ratatouille is particularly great for digestion and immunity.

1. Preheat the oven to 400°F. Lightly grease a 9-by-13-inch baking dish.

2. Put the zucchini, onion, eggplant, and tomatoes in a large bowl. Add the garlic, olive oil, salt, and herb mix. Toss to coat.

3. Transfer the mixture to the baking dish and roast until the vegetables are tender and lightly browned around the edges, 30 to 40 minutes.

4. Serve warm. Store leftovers in an airtight container in the refrigerator for up to 5 days.

PER SERVING: Calories: 160; Total fat: 8g; Sodium: 253mg; Carbohydrates: 22g; Fiber: 8g; Protein: 5g

# Simple Sautéed Greens

**5**

**30**

**OP**

**V**

SERVES: 4  |  PREP TIME: **5 Minutes**  |  COOK TIME: **10 Minutes**

SYMPTOMS: Fatigue / Anemia / Constipation

2 tablespoons extra-virgin
  olive oil

2 or 3 garlic cloves, minced
  or pressed

1 large shallot, minced

1 large bunch fresh kale
  or chard, stemmed and
  roughly chopped

1 (10-ounce) bag fresh
  spinach, stemmed and
  roughly chopped

Sea salt

Freshly ground black pepper

Pinch red pepper
  flakes (optional)

Dark, leafy greens are an important part of a cancer-healing diet. They are rich in iron and B vitamins, making them helpful in boosting red blood cell production. They are also a great source of fiber, carotenoids, and other phyto-nutrients. You can enjoy raw greens in salads, fresh juices, or smoothies, and cooked greens in soups or stews. I also like them on their own, simply sautéed. Feel free to use any leafy green you like in this recipe.

1. In a large skillet, heat the olive oil over medium heat until shimmering. Add the garlic and shallot and sauté for 1 minute or so, until fragrant.

2. Add the kale and stir, cooking until just tender, 4 to 5 minutes. Add the spinach and cook until wilted but still bright green, 1 to 2 minutes.

3. Season with salt and pepper and sprinkle on the red pepper flakes, if using. Serve immediately.

PER SERVING: Calories: 92; Total fat: 7g; Sodium: 105mg; Carbohydrates: 6g; Fiber: 3g; Protein: 3g

# Savory Sweet Potato Puree

| SERVES: 6 | PREP TIME: 10 Minutes | COOK TIME: 15 Minutes |

SYMPTOMS: Nausea / Trouble Swallowing / Taste Changes / Sore Mouth or Throat / Unintentional Weight Loss / Constipation

4 pounds sweet potatoes (about 6 medium), peeled and cut into 1-inch cubes

2 teaspoons sea salt, divided

¼ cup broth, preferably Mineral-Rich Bone Broth (page 160) or Basic Chicken Bone Broth (page 162)

3 tablespoons unsalted butter (preferably grass-fed), cut into cubes

⅓ cup thinly sliced scallion greens (from 1 bunch)

⅓ cup finely chopped fresh flat-leaf parsley

1 garlic clove, minced or pressed

Freshly ground black pepper

This recipe elevates traditional mashed potatoes to give you more fiber, flavor, and cancer-healing nutrients. While sweet potatoes are my favorite tuber for this dish, you can cook just about any root vegetable or gourd you like in this style: carrots, winter squash, turnips, parsnips, or beets. You may have noticed I prefer butter made from the milk of grass-fed cows. That's because compared to conventional butter, it has higher concentrations of healthy omega-3 fatty acids and conjugated linoleic acid, and it contains higher amounts of vitamin $K_2$ and beta-carotene.

1.  Place the sweet potatoes in a Dutch oven or large saucepan and add enough water to cover by about 1 inch. Add 1 teaspoon of the salt and bring to a boil over medium-high heat. Reduce the heat and simmer, uncovered, until the potatoes are tender, about 10 minutes.

2.  Drain, then return the potatoes to the pot. Add the broth and butter and puree with an immersion blender (or blend the ingredients in a food processor or blender, or mash by hand).

3. Stir in the scallions and parsley, reserving a bit for garnish, if you wish. Stir in the garlic, remaining 1 teaspoon of salt, and pepper to taste.

4. Serve promptly. Store leftovers in an airtight container in the refrigerator for 4 to 5 days.

PER SERVING: Calories: 316; Total fat: 6g; Sodium: 413mg; Carbohydrates: 62g; Fiber: 10g; Protein: 5g

# Kale Salad

SERVES: **4** | PREP TIME: **10 Minutes** | ///////////

SYMPTOMS: Nausea / Fatigue / Anemia / Taste Changes / Constipation

Juice of 1 large lemon
½ cup extra-virgin olive oil
2 garlic cloves, minced
  or pressed
¼ teaspoon sea salt
⅛ teaspoon freshly ground
  black pepper
1 bunch dinosaur
  kale, stemmed and
  roughly chopped
¼ cup pumpkin seeds

PREP AHEAD TIP: The best part about this salad is that the longer it sits in the fridge, the better it tastes. It's also easy to double the recipe to make a larger batch that you can eat throughout the week. Because it holds up so well, it's a great candidate for potlucks or barbecues.

I dare say this is the best kale salad you'll find, and it's one of my go-to ways to get more greens into my diet. It has become a favorite of many friends and clients, as well. It's simple to make, but the massaging technique makes all the difference between having a delicious, sweet, and tender salad and one that's bitter and hard to chew. To prepare the kale, use a knife to cut the leaves away from the stems and then roughly chop them, or just rip the leaves from the stems and tear them into pieces with your hands.

1. In a large salad bowl, whisk together the lemon juice, olive oil, garlic, salt, and pepper. Add the kale and massage with the dressing, squeezing and pinching with your hands, until the leaves are wilted, 3 to 4 minutes. (This is a critical step in making kale salad tender, so don't rush it—the longer you massage it, the better it will be.)

2. Top with the pumpkin seeds and serve immediately, or store in an airtight container in the refrigerator for up to 7 days.

PER SERVING: Calories: 298; Total fat: 30g; Sodium: 128mg; Carbohydrates: 5g; Fiber: 1g; Protein: 3g

# Rainbow Slaw

SERVES: 4        |        PREP TIME: 15 Minutes

SYMPTOMS: Fatigue / Anemia / Taste Changes / Constipation

Grated zest and juice of
1 large lemon
1 large shallot, finely chopped
2 teaspoons Dijon mustard
2 tablespoons jarred
capers, rinsed, drained,
and chopped
½ teaspoon sea salt
¼ teaspoon freshly ground
black pepper
¼ cup extra-virgin olive oil
1 pound Brussels sprouts,
trimmed and shredded
3 cups shredded purple
cabbage (about ⅓ head)
½ cup chopped almonds

Not only is this colorful slaw tasty and easy to make, but it's also full of fiber and anticancer phytonutrients. For the best and quickest results, shred the Brussels sprouts and cabbage in a food processor.

1. In a small bowl, whisk together the lemon zest and juice, shallot, mustard, capers, salt, and pepper. Pour in the oil in a steady stream and whisk to combine.

2. Place the shredded sprouts and cabbage in a large bowl. Pour the dressing over the vegetables and toss until well coated. (I like to do this with my hands.)

3. Sprinkle with the chopped almonds.

4. Serve. Store leftovers in an airtight container in the refrigerator for up to 4 days.

PER SERVING: Calories: 274; Total fat: 21g; Sodium: 408mg; Carbohydrates: 20g; Fiber: 8g; Protein: 8g

# Tomato and Basil Salad

SERVES: 4 | PREP TIME: 5 Minutes

SYMPTOMS: Fatigue / Anemia / Taste Changes

1 pint cherry tomatoes, halved

1 (8-ounce) container small mozzarella balls, halved

2 garlic cloves, minced or pressed

¼ cup chopped fresh basil

2 tablespoons extra-virgin olive oil

Pinch sea salt

Drizzle balsamic vinegar (optional)

There is nothing like the taste of a good summer tomato. And when it's paired with olive oil, garlic, and basil, it is summertime magic. Tomatoes are a great source of vitamin C, antioxidants, potassium, and anti-cancer phytonutrients. The most notable of these phytonutrients is lycopene, which is particularly important in helping prevent prostate cancer. Add the garlic and basil, and this recipe is a great immunity supporter.

Combine the tomatoes, mozzarella, garlic, basil, olive oil, salt, and vinegar, if using, in a large bowl. Toss well, then serve. Store leftovers in an airtight container in the refrigerator for 2 to 3 days, and be aware that the basil will darken.

PER SERVING: Calories: 239; Total fat: 20g; Sodium: 397mg; Carbohydrates: 3g; Fiber: 1g; Protein: 13g

# Walnut, Pear, and Pomegranate Salad

**30**

**OP**

**VG**

SERVES: **4** | PREP TIME: **10 Minutes**

SYMPTOMS: Fatigue / Anemia / Taste Changes / Constipation

1 cup raw walnut halves

¼ cup Balsamic Vinaigrette (page 167)

1 (12-ounce) bag mixed fresh greens

1 cup pomegranate seeds (from 1 pomegranate)

2 ripe pears (such as Anjou, Comice, or Bartlett), cored and thinly sliced

1 (4-ounce) container crumbled goat cheese (chèvre)

An irresistible combination of sweet, tangy, crunchy, and creamy ingredients, this salad has been on our Thanksgiving table for years. The walnuts and goat cheese add protein and healthy fat, while the pears and pomegranates contribute more fiber, vitamin C, folate, potassium, and antioxidants, as well as anti-inflammatory and anticancer phytonutrients.

1. In a dry skillet over medium-high heat, lightly toast the walnuts, stirring until fragrant, 2 to 3 minutes.

2. Pour the dressing into a large salad bowl, then add the walnuts, greens, pomegranate seeds, pears, and goat cheese. Toss to coat and serve.

PER SERVING: Calories: 374; Total fat: 26g; Sodium: 241mg; Carbohydrates: 30g; Fiber: 7g; Protein: 12g

# Warm Beet, Feta, and Mint Salad

| SERVES: 4 | PREP TIME: 10 Minutes | COOK TIME: 30 Minutes |

SYMPTOMS: Fatigue / Anemia / Taste Changes / Constipation

4 medium beets, peeled and cut into 1½-inch cubes

1 tablespoon extra-virgin olive oil or avocado oil

¼ teaspoon sea salt

¼ cup Balsamic Vinaigrette (page 167)

½ cup crumbled feta cheese

2 tablespoons roughly chopped fresh mint

Beets are a great cancer-healing food. They are a good source of fiber, as well as anti-inflammatory and anticancer phytonutrients. Feta provides protein and healthy fat, and the pairing is a classic sweet-salty combination. If you have roasted beets on hand in the refrigerator, this salad will take only 5 minutes to pull together.

1. Preheat the oven to 400°F. Line a baking sheet with parchment paper.

2. Put the beets on the baking sheet and drizzle with the olive oil. Sprinkle with the salt, toss to coat, and spread out in a single layer. Roast until the beets are tender and slightly browned, 25 to 30 minutes.

3. Pour the dressing into a large salad bowl. Add the beets, feta, and mint. Toss together to coat.

4. Serve immediately. Store leftovers in an airtight container in the refrigerator for up to 4 days.

MAKE IT EASIER TIP: Some grocery stores sell vacuum-packed boiled beets, or you can boil fresh beets yourself, then peel and cube them, instead of roasting the beets.

PER SERVING: Calories: 142; Total fat: 8g; Sodium: 467mg; Carbohydrates: 15g; Fiber: 4g; Protein: 5g

# Nourish Bowl

SERVES: **2** | PREP TIME: **10 Minutes**

SYMPTOMS: Fatigue / Anemia / Constipation

4 cups salad greens

1 cup diced roasted
  sweet potato

1 cup cherry tomatoes

½ cup broccoli sprouts

1 avocado, pitted, peeled,
  and sliced

2 hard-boiled eggs, halved

2 tablespoons Balsamic
  Vinaigrette (page 167)

There is no wrong way to build a nourish bowl. As long as you have a balanced mix of greens, colorful vegetables, starch, protein, and healthy fat, you can be as creative as you want. Try to add as many colorful vegetables, either raw or cooked, as you can and don't be afraid to throw in some fermented or pickled veggies, too. Choose a whole grain (wild rice, quinoa, farro, barley) or starchy vegetable (roasted sweet potato, squash). The protein can be plant- or animal-based (such as beans, lentils, chicken, salmon, tuna, eggs, nuts, or seeds). And my favorite fats include avocado, nuts, seeds, olives, and homemade dressing (see chapter 8). This is one of my favorite combinations.

Divide the salad greens, sweet potato, tomatoes, sprouts, avocado slices, and eggs between 2 bowls, top with the dressing, and serve.

PER SERVING: Calories: 355; Total fat: 22g; Sodium: 294mg; Carbohydrates: 34g; Fiber: 13g; Protein: 13g

# Quinoa and Black Bean Salad

SERVES: 4 | PREP TIME: 10 Minutes | COOK TIME: 20 Minutes

SYMPTOMS: Fatigue / Trouble Swallowing / Anemia / Diarrhea / Constipation

2 cups vegetable broth (such as Mineral-Rich Vegetable Broth, page 158), or water

1 cup quinoa, rinsed

1 tablespoon extra-virgin olive oil

½ medium onion, finely chopped

½ red bell pepper, finely chopped

1 medium carrot, finely chopped

1 teaspoon chili powder

½ teaspoon ground cumin

¼ teaspoon sea salt

¼ cup Lime-Garlic Dressing (see variation, page 168)

1 (15-ounce) can black beans, rinsed and drained

3 scallions, white and green parts, thinly sliced

1 celery stalk, finely chopped

½ cup fresh cilantro, roughly chopped

Quinoa has the highest protein content of all grains and is naturally gluten-free. The black beans are a good source of iron and calcium, as well as magnesium and antioxidants. This flavorful salad can be made ahead of time and stored in an airtight container in the refrigerator for up to 4 days.

1. Bring the broth and quinoa to a boil in a large, deep pot or Dutch oven over medium-high heat. Reduce the heat to low and simmer, covered, for 15 to 20 minutes, until the quinoa has absorbed all the liquid. Spread the quinoa evenly on a baking sheet and let it cool.

2. Meanwhile, heat the olive oil in a small skillet over medium heat. Add the onion and cook until translucent, about 2 minutes. Add the bell pepper and carrot and cook until tender, another 2 minutes. Add the chili powder, cumin, and salt and cook until fragrant, about 2 minutes more.

3. Pour the dressing into a large bowl. Add the quinoa, onion mixture, beans, scallions, celery, and cilantro. Toss together well. Serve at room temperature.

PER SERVING: Calories: 381; Total fat: 16g; Sodium: 177mg; Carbohydrates: 48g; Fiber: 10g; Protein: 13g

# Simple Tabbouleh

| SERVES: 4 | PREP TIME: 5 Minutes | COOK TIME: 15 Minutes |

SYMPTOMS: Fatigue / Anemia / Taste Changes / Constipation

2 cups vegetable broth (such as Mineral-Rich Vegetable Broth, page 158), or water

1 cup bulgur

¼ cup Lemon-Garlic Dressing (page 168)

2 cups finely chopped fresh flat-leaf parsley

¼ cup fresh mint leaves, finely chopped

2 ripe medium tomatoes, diced

1 small cucumber, seeded and diced

4 scallions, white and green parts, thinly sliced

VARIATION TIP: For gluten-free tabbouleh, substitute quinoa for the bulgur. To make the quinoa, combine the broth and 1 cup of quinoa in a medium saucepan. Bring to a boil over high heat, then reduce the heat to low and simmer, covered, for 15 to 20 minutes, until all the liquid is absorbed. Spread the quinoa on a baking sheet, rake with a fork, and let it cool.

Bulgur is a whole grain and a great source of fiber, B vitamins, and minerals like manganese, magnesium, and iron. It supports a healthy gut and balanced blood sugar. Parsley is a good source of antioxidants, like vitamins A and C, as well as folate and potassium. This herb also contains anticancer and detox-supporting phytonutrients. To make the prep a bit easier, you can use a food processor to help you chop the parsley and mint.

1. In a medium saucepan, combine the broth and bulgur. Bring to a boil over high heat, cover, and reduce the heat to low. Simmer until tender, about 15 minutes. Drain off any excess liquid and fluff with a fork.

2. Pour the dressing into a large bowl, then add the bulgur. Stir in the parsley, mint, tomatoes, cucumber, and scallions. Toss together well.

3. Serve at room temperature. The tabbouleh can be stored in an airtight container in the refrigerator for up to 4 days.

PER SERVING: Calories: 241; Total fat: 10g; Sodium: 49mg; Carbohydrates: 35g; Fiber: 7g; Protein: 7g

# Spring Greens with Spiced Chickpeas

| SERVES: 4 | PREP TIME: 5 Minutes | COOK TIME: 20 Minutes |

SYMPTOMS: Fatigue / Anemia / Taste Changes / Constipation

1 teaspoon smoked paprika

1 teaspoon ground cumin

¾ teaspoon sea salt, divided

¼ teaspoon cayenne

¾ cup plus 1 tablespoon avocado oil or other high-smoke-point oil, divided

1½ cups cooked chickpeas, or 1 (15-ounce) can chickpeas, rinsed, drained, and thoroughly dried

1 red onion, halved and thinly sliced

6 ounces fresh spring greens or mesclun mix

¼ cup Honey Mustard Dressing (page 169)

The chickpeas in this tasty salad are full of protein, fiber, B vitamins, and iron, and the dressing and oil provide healthy fat. Meanwhile, the leafy greens and spices offer an assortment of anticancer nutrients. To add more calories to this salad, drizzle on a bit more dressing and add sliced avocado.

1. In a large bowl, combine the paprika, cumin, ½ teaspoon of the salt, and the cayenne.

2. In a Dutch oven, heat ¾ cup of oil over high heat until shimmering. Add the chickpeas, partially cover to prevent splattering, and cook, stirring occasionally, until the chickpeas are a deep golden brown and crispy, about 10 minutes.

3. Using a slotted spoon, transfer the chickpeas to a paper towel–lined plate and let them drain briefly. Toss the chickpeas in the bowl with the spices.

4. To caramelize the onion, adjust the oven rack 6 inches from the broiler and preheat the broiler. Line a baking sheet with parchment paper.

5. Toss the onion with the 1 tablespoon of oil and the remaining ¼ teaspoon of salt and spread on the baking sheet. Broil the onion until its edges are charred, 6 to 8 minutes, stirring halfway through cooking.

6. Let the onion cool slightly, then add to the bowl along with the salad greens. Drizzle the dressing over and toss to combine. Serve immediately.

PREP AHEAD TIP: You can make the spiced chickpeas ahead of time and store them in an airtight container in the refrigerator for up to 5 days (they also make a great snack).

PER SERVING: Calories: 189; Total fat: 11g; Sodium: 438mg; Carbohydrates: 16g; Fiber: 4g; Protein: 5g

# French Lentil Salad

SERVES: 6 | PREP: **10 Minutes** | COOK: **20 to 30 Minutes**

SYMPTOMS: Nausea / Fatigue / Anemia / Diarrhea

2 cups French green or
 black lentils

1 dried bay leaf

2 teaspoons herbes
 de Provence

1 strip kombu
 (3 to 4 inches)

½ red onion, diced

2 cups fresh arugula or other
 salad green

½ cup chopped raw walnuts

⅓ cup extra-virgin olive oil

Juice of 1 lemon

2 garlic cloves, minced
 or pressed

2 teaspoons Dijon mustard

½ teaspoon sea salt

¼ teaspoon freshly ground
 black pepper

Lentils are the star of this protein- and fiber-packed salad. These legumes are easier to digest than other beans, and adding the strip of kombu, a type of seaweed, helps make them even more digestible. If you can't find kombu, don't worry; you can still make these lentils without it. There are many different kinds of lentils to choose from. I prefer French green lentils (also known as lentils du Puy) and black lentils, but most all lentils will work here, other than red lentils, which become really soft and almost like a puree when cooked.

1.  Rinse the lentils in a fine-mesh sieve. Inspect the lentils and remove any bad ones or small stones.

2.  Place the lentils in a large pot and cover with water by 2 inches. Add the bay leaf, herbes de Provence, and kombu. Bring to a boil, reduce the heat to very low, cover, and simmer for 25 to 30 minutes, or until the lentils are tender but not mushy.

3.  Drain the lentils, remove the bay leaf and kombu, and transfer the lentils to a large mixing bowl.

4. Add the onion, arugula, and walnuts and stir to combine. (The salad, without the dressing, can be stored in an airtight container in the refrigerator for up to 1 week.)

5. When ready to serve, in a small mixing bowl, whisk together the olive oil, lemon juice, garlic, mustard, salt, and pepper. Drizzle over the salad and toss to combine.

PREP AHEAD TIP: Lentils are a good protein option to make ahead, store in the refrigerator, and then add to different meals. It's a quick, easy-to-digest, and tasty protein that can be added to salads, soups, or even atop a cooked sweet potato.

PER SERVING: Calories: 404; Total fat: 19g; Sodium: 180mg; Carbohydrates: 44g; Fiber: 8g; Protein: 18g

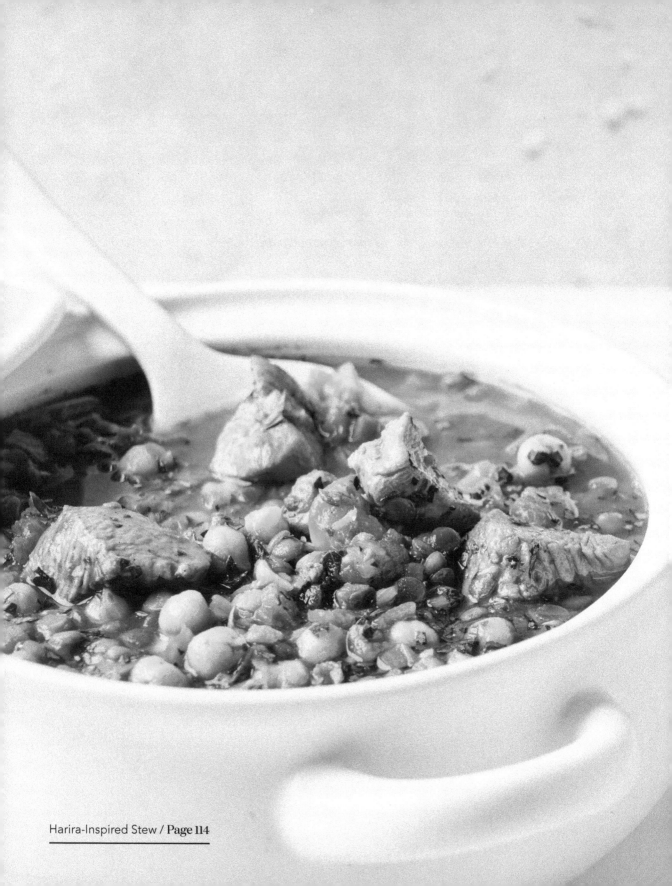

Harira-Inspired Stew / Page 114

# CHAPTER 5

# Soothing Soups

# Roasted Butternut Squash, Apple, and Sage Soup

| SERVES: 4 | PREP TIME: 10 Minutes | COOK TIME: 50 Minutes |

SYMPTOMS: Nausea / Trouble Swallowing / Taste Changes / Sore Mouth or Throat / Unintentional Weight Loss / Diarrhea / Constipation

1 large butternut squash (3 to 4 pounds), halved lengthwise, seeds removed

2 large shallots, quartered

2 medium to large apples, peeled, cored, and quartered

1 (1-inch) piece of fresh ginger, peeled and cut into thirds

2 tablespoons extra-virgin olive oil

1 cup canned full-fat coconut milk

8 fresh sage leaves, or 1 tablespoon ground

½ teaspoon sea salt, or more as desired

Toasted pepitas or almond slices, for garnish (optional)

Unlike most hearty soup recipes, this one doesn't require any stovetop time. Simply roast all your veggies in the oven, then blend with coconut milk and sage. The squash and apples are good sources of fiber, as well as potassium, vitamin A, and other anticancer phytonutrients. Coconut milk is a great source of healthy fat and calories. And the shallots, ginger, and sage provide flavor and an immune boost.

1. Preheat the oven to 400°F. Line a baking sheet with parchment paper.

2. Place the squash cut side down on the baking sheet and add the shallots, apples, and ginger in a single layer. Drizzle with the olive oil and use your hands to coat the ingredients. Cover the baking sheet with a large piece of foil, sealing around the edges.

3. Roast until the apples are tender, about 30 minutes. Remove the apples from the baking sheet, along with the shallots and ginger. Reseal the baking sheet with the foil and roast the squash for another 20 minutes, or until soft enough to be easily pierced with a fork. Let it cool.

4. When cool enough to handle, scoop out the flesh from the squash and place in a food processor or high-speed blender. Add the apples, shallots, and ginger, then add the coconut milk, sage, and salt. Blend until smooth. If the mixture is too thick, add warm water a tablespoon at a time until you reach the desired consistency. Adjust the salt to taste.

5. Pour the soup into bowls and sprinkle with pepitas or almond slices, if using. Serve immediately. Store leftovers in an airtight container in the refrigerator for up to 1 week or in the freezer for up to 3 months.

FLAVOR BOOST TIP: When dealing with taste changes, you can enhance the flavor of this soup by adding more ginger or squeezing some fresh lime or lemon juice over the top just before serving.

PER SERVING: Calories: 367; Total fat: 19g; Sodium: 254mg; Carbohydrates: 53g; Fiber: 8g; Protein: 5g

# Pumpkin Curry Soup

| SERVES: 4 | PREP TIME: 5 Minutes | COOK TIME: 25 Minutes |

SYMPTOMS: Nausea / Trouble Swallowing / Taste Changes / Unintentional Weight Loss / Diarrhea

1 tablespoon unsalted butter (preferably grass-fed)

1 large onion, chopped

2 garlic cloves, minced or pressed

2 teaspoons peeled and minced fresh ginger

1½ teaspoons curry powder

1 teaspoon ground cumin

½ teaspoon ground coriander

½ teaspoon ground cinnamon

½ teaspoon sea salt

4 cups vegetable broth (such as Mineral-Rich Vegetable Broth, page 158)

2 dried bay leaves

2 (15-ounce) cans pumpkin puree

¼ cup heavy cream

Freshly ground black pepper

Toasted pepitas, for garnish

This comforting soup proves that pumpkins can be so much more than just a star ingredient in your holiday pie. They are an excellent source of vitamin A and carotenoids, and they also provide vitamin C, potassium, and fiber. Like carrots, they contain phytonutrients that support the immune system and lower inflammation. The garlic, ginger, and spices also boost immunity, lower inflammation, and provide anticancer nutrients—and they give this soup its incredible flavor.

1. In a Dutch oven or deep saucepan, heat the butter over medium heat. Add the onion and cook, stirring, until soft and translucent, about 5 minutes. Add the garlic and ginger and cook, stirring, for another minute. Stir in the curry, cumin, coriander, cinnamon, and salt and sauté for 2 minutes more.

2. Add the broth, bay leaves, and pumpkin puree to the Dutch oven. Stir to combine, increase the heat to high, and bring to a boil. Reduce to low and simmer, covered, for 15 minutes.

3. Remove the bay leaves and puree the soup with an immersion blender (or in a blender, working in batches). Stir in the cream and add pepper to taste.

4. Serve warm, topped with toasted pumpkin seeds, if using. Store leftovers in an airtight container in the refrigerator for up to 1 week or in the freezer for up to 3 months.

VARIATION TIPS: Make this recipe dairy-free by substituting coconut oil for the butter and coconut cream for the heavy cream. If preferred, use roasted fresh pumpkin instead of canned puree. To roast the pumpkin, preheat the oven to 350°F. Line a baking sheet with parchment paper. Cut a pumpkin in half and place the halves cut side down on the baking sheet. Bake for about 1 hour, until the flesh is soft enough to be easily pierced with a fork. Let the pumpkin cool. Scoop out the flesh and measure 3½ cups for the soup.

PER SERVING: Calories: 200; Total fat: 9g; Sodium: 376mg; Carbohydrates: 31g; Fiber: 3g; Protein: 4g

# Spiced Squash Soup

SERVES: 6 to 8 | PREP TIME: 10 Minutes | COOK TIME: 35 Minutes

SYMPTOMS: Nausea / Fatigue / Trouble Swallowing / Taste Changes / Diarrhea

2 tablespoons extra-virgin olive oil

1 medium onion, diced

½ teaspoon sea salt, divided

½ teaspoon ground ginger

¼ teaspoon ground cinnamon

¼ teaspoon ground cardamom

¼ teaspoon chili powder

¼ teaspoon ground nutmeg

3 large carrots, cut into small chunks

1 large parsnip, peeled and cut into small chunks

1 large winter squash (about 3 pounds), peeled, seeded, and cut into small chunks

¼ teaspoon dried thyme

3 garlic cloves, minced or pressed

1 (2-inch) piece of fresh ginger, peeled and minced

6 to 8 cups vegetable broth (such as Mineral-Rich Vegetable Broth, page 158)

Any winter squash will work well in this recipe, but I like to use kabocha or pumpkin. The vegetables provide a good dose of fiber plus antioxidants, digestive support, and immune-boosting nutrients. The spices, onion, garlic, and fresh ginger are all great anticancer, anti-inflammatory, and immune-boosting foods. Creamy squash and root vegetables are naturally sweet and comforting, and can be just the answer when you don't feel like eating.

1. Heat the olive oil in a Dutch oven or large, deep pot over medium heat. Add the onion, ¼ teaspoon of the salt, the ground ginger, cinnamon, cardamom, chili powder, and nutmeg and sauté until the onion is translucent, about 3 minutes. Add the carrots, parsnip, and squash, stir to combine, and cook until the vegetables begin to brown and soften, about 10 minutes. Add the remaining ¼ teaspoon of salt along with the thyme, garlic, and fresh ginger and stir to combine.

2. Add 6 cups of the broth and stir to combine. Bring to a boil, then reduce the heat to medium-low and cover. Cook for approximately 20 minutes, until the vegetables are tender.

3. Puree the soup with an immersion blender (or in a blender, working in batches) until smooth and creamy, adding more broth as needed to achieve your preferred consistency.

4. Serve warm. Store leftovers in an airtight container in the refrigerator for up to 1 week or in the freezer for up to 3 months.

PER SERVING: Calories: 174; Total fat: 5g; Sodium: 241mg; Carbohydrates: 34g; Fiber: 6g; Protein: 3g

# Potato, Leek, and Cauliflower Soup

| SERVES: 6 | PREP TIME: 5 Minutes | COOK TIME: 25 Minutes |

**SYMPTOMS:** Nausea / Fatigue / Trouble Swallowing / Anemia / Sore Mouth or Throat / Unintentional Weight Loss / Constipation

1½ cups unsweetened almond or coconut milk

½ head cauliflower, cored and roughly chopped (about 4 cups)

2 tablespoons extra-virgin olive oil

2 leeks, light green and white parts only, thinly sliced

3 garlic cloves, minced or pressed

4 cups vegetable broth (such as Mineral-Rich Vegetable Broth, page 158)

2 russet potatoes (about 1 pound), peeled and cut into chunks

2 dried bay leaves

½ teaspoon dried rosemary, crushed to release oils

½ teaspoon sea salt, or more as needed

½ teaspoon freshly ground black pepper, or more as needed

A vegan riff on vichyssoise, this soup highlights one of my favorite anticancer vegetables: cauliflower. In addition to being a great source of fiber, cauliflower is full of vitamin C, B vitamins, and phytonutrients that support detoxification and hormone balance. I like to use rosemary in this recipe, but it would also work well with other dried herbs, like thyme or sage.

1. In a medium saucepan, combine the almond milk and cauliflower. Cook over medium-high heat until the cauliflower is tender and a fork pierces it easily, about 5 minutes.

2. In a Dutch oven or large, deep pot, heat the olive oil over medium-high heat until shimmering. Add the leeks and cook until softened, about 8 minutes. Add the garlic and cook until fragrant, about 30 seconds. Add the broth, potatoes, bay leaves, rosemary, salt, and pepper and bring to a simmer. Cook until the potatoes are tender, about 10 minutes.

3. Remove the bay leaves and add the cauliflower mixture. Puree with an immersion blender (or in a blender, working in batches). Adjust the salt and pepper to taste.

4. Serve warm. Store leftovers in an airtight container in the refrigerator for up to 1 week or in the freezer for up to 3 months.

PER SERVING: Calories: 208; Total fat: 5g; Sodium: 252mg; Carbohydrates: 37g; Fiber: 3g; Protein: 4g

# Moroccan-Inspired Vegetable Soup with Chickpeas

SERVES: 6 | PREP TIME: 10 Minutes | COOK TIME: 25 Minutes

SYMPTOMS: Fatigue / Trouble Swallowing / Anemia / Taste Changes / Sore Mouth or Throat / Diarrhea

2 tablespoons extra-virgin olive oil

1 large onion, chopped

2 celery stalks, chopped

1 medium sweet potato, peeled and cut into ½-inch cubes

1 large carrot, diced

2 large garlic cloves, minced or pressed

1½ teaspoons ground cumin

1 teaspoon ground turmeric

½ teaspoon ground coriander

½ teaspoon ground cinnamon

½ teaspoon sea salt

¼ teaspoon freshly ground black pepper

Pinch saffron

6 cups vegetable broth (such as Mineral-Rich Vegetable Broth, page 158)

2 (15-ounce) cans chickpeas, rinsed and drained

1 lemon, cut into wedges

One of the things I love most about Moroccan food is the variety of spices—such as turmeric, cinnamon, cumin, coriander, and ground ginger—that are essential to so many recipes. They not only provide delicious flavor but also contain phytonutrients that can boost the immune system, lower inflammation, and help the body fight off cancer. This spicy, vitamin-rich soup is a great recipe to make ahead of time and enjoy over the course of the week.

1. In a Dutch oven or large, deep pot, heat the oil over medium heat. Add the onion and celery and sauté until golden, about 6 minutes. Add the sweet potato and carrot and sauté until starting to soften, another 3 minutes. Stir in the garlic, cumin, turmeric, coriander, cinnamon, salt, pepper, and saffron and cook for another minute.

2. Pour in ½ cup of the broth to deglaze the pot, stirring and scraping with a wooden spoon to get up the browned bits. Add the chickpeas and the remaining 5½ cups of broth. Bring to a boil, reduce the heat to low, cover, and simmer until the vegetables are soft, about 15 minutes.

3. Puree the soup with an immersion blender (or in a blender, working in batches). I enjoy this soup partially pureed, with some pieces of vegetables and chickpeas still whole.

4. Serve warm with a squeeze of fresh lemon juice. Store leftovers in an airtight container in the refrigerator for up to 1 week or in the freezer for up to 3 months.

FLAVOR BOOST TIP: Add a refreshing burst of flavor with a sprinkle of chopped fresh cilantro or mint.

PER SERVING: Calories: 256; Total fat: 8g; Sodium: 421mg; Carbohydrates: 38g; Fiber: 10g; Protein: 10g

# Mushroom Barley Soup

**SERVES: 4** | **PREP TIME: 25 Minutes** | **COOK TIME: 45 Minutes**

**SYMPTOMS:** Nausea / Fatigue / Trouble Swallowing / Anemia / Sore Mouth or Throat / Diarrhea / Constipation

½ ounce dried
 porcini mushrooms

½ ounce dried
 shiitake mushrooms

4 cups boiling water

3 tablespoons extra-virgin
 olive oil

1 medium onion, diced

12 ounces fresh cremini
 or white button
 mushrooms, sliced

1 carrot, diced

1 celery stalk, sliced

2 garlic cloves, minced
 or pressed

1 teaspoon dried thyme, or
 1 tablespoon minced fresh

4 cups vegetable broth (such
 as Mineral-Rich Vegetable
 Broth, page 158)

½ cup pearl barley

1 teaspoon sea salt

½ teaspoon freshly ground
 black pepper

The blend of mushrooms in this soup offers rich flavor and a variety of anticancer nutrients. Barley is an ancient whole grain that is rich in nutrients and soluble fiber, and it has a low glycemic index. The combination of barley and mushrooms provides a fair amount of protein to this vegan soup. Barley does contain gluten, so if you're gluten-free, substitute a gluten-free grain, such as oat groats or brown or wild rice.

1. Place the porcini and shiitake mushrooms in a medium bowl and pour the boiling water over. Cover with plastic wrap or a plate and let soak for 20 minutes. Strain the mushrooms through a fine-mesh sieve over a bowl and reserve the liquid. Finely chop the mushrooms.

2. In a Dutch oven or large, deep pot, heat the olive oil over medium-high heat. Add the onion and cook for about 4 minutes, until translucent. Stir in the cremini mushrooms, carrot, and celery and cook until tender, 5 to 6 minutes. Add the garlic and thyme, stir to combine, and cook until fragrant, about 30 seconds more.

3. Add ½ cup of the broth to deglaze the pot, stirring and scraping with a wooden spoon to get up the browned bits. Stir until the liquid is reduced by half, about 3 minutes. Add the soaked mushrooms, reserved mushroom water, remaining 3½ cups of broth, barley, salt, and pepper. Bring to a simmer, reduce the heat to low, and cook for 35 to 40 minutes, until the barley is tender.

4. Serve warm. Store leftovers in an airtight container in the refrigerator for up to 1 week or in the freezer for up to 3 months. I think this soup tastes even better after a few days.

MAKE IT EASIER TIP: You can cook the barley ahead of time and store in the refrigerator for up to 5 days. This will bring down the cooking time considerably. At step 4 you can add the cooked barley, bring to a simmer, and cook for just another 10 minutes to heat through and allow the flavors to meld.

PER SERVING: Calories: 238; Total fat: 11g; Sodium: 488mg; Carbohydrates: 32g; Fiber: 7g; Protein: 6g

# Black Bean Soup

| SERVES: 4 | PREP TIME: 10 Minutes | COOK TIME: 20 Minutes |

SYMPTOMS: Nausea / Fatigue / Trouble Swallowing / Anemia / Sore Mouth or Throat / Diarrhea

2 tablespoons extra-virgin olive oil

1 medium onion, finely chopped

1 celery stalk, diced

2 garlic cloves, minced or pressed

1½ teaspoons dry mustard

¼ teaspoon ground cloves

5 cups vegetable broth (such as Mineral-Rich Vegetable Broth, page 158)

3 (15-ounce) cans black beans, rinsed and drained

2 dried bay leaves

½ teaspoon sea salt, or more as needed

1 cup crème fraîche or plain full-fat Greek yogurt

Freshly ground black pepper

1 avocado, pitted, peeled, and diced

Black beans are an excellent source of fiber and protein, and they also provide food for the good bacteria in your gut, making them important for digestive health. These legumes can be especially effective at slowing down digestion and bulking up loose or watery stool. If you're not used to eating beans, they may be a bit hard to digest, but soaking them overnight, cooking them long enough, and using kombu (a type of seaweed) during cooking will all improve their digestibility. If you're using canned beans, look for brands that cook their beans in this way, such as Eden Foods.

1. In a Dutch oven or large, deep pot, heat the oil over medium heat, then add the onion, celery, and garlic. Cook for about 3 minutes, stirring occasionally, until the onion is translucent.

2. Stir in the mustard and cloves. Add 1 cup of the broth and simmer until the onion is softened, about 2 minutes. Then add the beans, another 3 cups of the broth, bay leaves, and salt. Cook until heated through and fragrant, about 15 minutes.

3. Remove the soup from the heat, discard the bay leaves, and puree with an immersion blender (or in a blender, working in batches) until smooth and creamy. Add more broth, if needed, to achieve your desired consistency. Stir in the crème fraîche and season to taste with salt and pepper.

4. Serve warm, topped with the avocado. Store leftovers in an airtight container in the refrigerator for up to 1 week or in the freezer for up to 3 months.

FLAVOR BOOST TIP: Squeeze a fresh lemon or lime over the top, sprinkle with minced fresh parsley or cilantro, or top with chopped jalapeños or a squirt of hot sauce.

PER SERVING: Calories: 430; Total fat: 17g; Sodium: 290mg; Carbohydrates: 53g; Fiber: 20g; Protein: 20g

# Miso Soup with Tofu and Greens

**SERVES:** 4 to 6 | **PREP TIME:** 5 Minutes | **COOK TIME:** 10 Minutes

**SYMPTOMS:** Nausea / Fatigue / Trouble Swallowing / Sore Mouth or Throat / Diarrhea

8 cups Basic Fish Broth (page 166) or Mineral-Rich Vegetable Broth (page 158)

3 tablespoons dried wakame, or 2 sheets nori, torn or cut into 1½-inch squares

4 tablespoons miso paste, preferably white or yellow

¼ cup hot water

1 cup chopped fresh chard, spinach, or other leafy green

1 cup chopped scallions, white and green parts

8 ounces firm tofu, cut into bite-size cubes

1 cup fresh mushrooms (such as shiitake or portobello), sliced (optional)

Sea salt (optional)

Miso, a fermented soybean paste, is a great source of easy-to-digest protein and probiotics that supports digestive health. It contains many other nutrients, including zinc, copper, vitamin K, and manganese. The phytoestrogens in both miso and tofu are good for hormone balance. Tofu is also a great source of protein. The seaweed in this soup adds essential minerals, like iodine, zinc, and iron, as well as nutrients to support detoxification. The greens and mushrooms boost the nutritional density even more. Miso is naturally high in sodium, so you can probably skip the salt in this recipe. Also be mindful that not all miso is gluten-free. Check the label if you're following a gluten-free diet.

1. In a Dutch oven or large, deep pot, bring the broth to a simmer over low heat. Add the wakame and simmer for 5 to 7 minutes. (If you're using nori, wait until the end of step 3 to add.)

2. Place the miso in a small bowl, add the hot water, and whisk until smooth. This ensures the miso will not clump when added to the soup.

3.  Add the chard, scallion, tofu, and mushrooms, if using, to the pot and cook until the vegetables are soft and the chard is wilted, about 5 minutes. Remove from the heat, add the miso mixture, and stir to combine. Taste and add more miso or a pinch of sea salt, if needed. (Add the nori, if using.)

4.  Serve at once, as this soup is best eaten the day it is made.

PER SERVING: Calories: 112; Total fat: 5.5g; Sodium: 779mg; Carbohydrates: 9g; Fiber: 3g; Protein: 10g

OP

V

# Aromatic Lentil Soup

| SERVES: 8 | PREP TIME: 10 Minutes | COOK TIME: 45 Minutes |

SYMPTOMS: Nausea / Fatigue / Trouble Swallowing / Anemia / Taste Changes / Diarrhea

Not only is this recipe flavorful and delicious, but it's also full of anticancer, anti-inflammatory, immune-boosting vegetables and spices. The lentils provide an easy-to-digest plant-based protein along with a healthy dose of fiber to support gut health. The lentils and spinach provide iron, while the vitamin C in the tomatoes helps increase the absorption of the iron, making this a great soup to support anemia and fatigue. The onions, carrots, garlic, cauliflower, and spices all provide an excellent dose of cancer-healing nutrition.

1 tablespoon extra-virgin olive oil

2 medium onions, chopped (about 2 cups)

2 large carrots, chopped (about 2 cups)

4 garlic cloves, minced or pressed

1 teaspoon ground cumin

1 teaspoon ground coriander

1 teaspoon ground turmeric

½ teaspoon ground cinnamon

½ teaspoon sea salt

¼ teaspoon freshly ground black pepper

8 cups vegetable broth (such as Mineral-Rich Vegetable Broth, page 158)

½ head cauliflower, cored and chopped

2 cups green or brown lentils, rinsed

1 (28-ounce) can diced tomatoes

2 tablespoons tomato paste

4 cups chopped fresh spinach, or 1 (10-ounce) package frozen spinach, thawed

Chopped fresh cilantro, for garnish

Fresh lemon juice

1. In a Dutch oven or large, deep pot, heat the oil over medium heat, then add the onions and carrots. Cook, stirring occasionally, until softened, about 10 minutes. Stir in the garlic and cook for about 30 seconds. Add the cumin, coriander, turmeric, cinnamon, salt, and pepper. Cook, stirring, until fragrant, about 1 minute.

2. Add the broth, cauliflower, lentils, tomatoes with their juice, and tomato paste, then increase the heat to high and bring to a boil. Reduce the heat to low, cover partially, and simmer until the lentils are tender but not mushy, 30 to 40 minutes. Stir in the spinach and cook until just wilted, 3 to 4 minutes.

3. Serve warm, sprinkled with cilantro and drizzled with lemon juice. Store leftovers in an airtight container in the refrigerator for up to 1 week or in the freezer for up to 3 months.

PER SERVING: Calories: 240; Total fat: 3g; Sodium: 273mg; Carbohydrates: 43g; Fiber: 10g; Protein: 15g

# Coconut Curry Soup with Shrimp

| SERVES: 4 | PREP TIME: 10 Minutes | COOK TIME: 15 Minutes |
|---|---|---|

SYMPTOMS: Fatigue / Anemia / Taste Changes

This bright and flavorful coconut curry soup contains anticancer veggies like carrots, broccoli, and leafy greens. The coconut milk provides healthy fat, while the shrimp provides protein. The shellfish in this soup is also a good source of zinc, selenium, iodine, and vitamin $B_{12}$, as well as antioxidants like astaxanthin. And although it may not be the first food that comes to mind when you think of omega-3 fatty acids, shrimp also contain these healthy fats.

1 tablespoon coconut oil

1 medium yellow or white onion, diced

1 red bell pepper, cored, seeded, and diced

1 large carrot, diced

1 cup chopped broccoli

3 garlic cloves, minced or pressed

1 tablespoon grated fresh ginger (from 1-inch piece)

2 tablespoons curry paste or curry powder

1 tablespoon soy sauce

1 (12-ounce) can full-fat coconut milk

4 cups Basic Fish Broth (page 166) or Mineral-Rich Vegetable Broth (page 158)

1 (12-ounce) package rice noodles

1 pound medium shrimp, peeled and deveined

2 cups chopped fresh spinach, chard, or other leafy green

⅓ cup chopped fresh cilantro, plus more for garnish (optional)

Juice of 1 lime

Hot sauce (optional)

Minced scallion greens, for garnish (optional)

Chopped fresh Thai basil, for garnish (optional)

1. In a Dutch oven or large, deep pot, heat the oil over medium-high heat. Add the onion and sauté for 1 minute. Add the bell pepper and carrot and cook for 1 minute more. Add the broccoli and cook until it starts to turn bright green, another 3 minutes. Stir in the garlic, ginger, curry paste, and soy sauce and cook for 30 seconds.

2. Add the coconut milk and broth and bring to a simmer, stirring occasionally, about 5 minutes. Add the noodles and shrimp and cook just until the shrimp turn pink, 3 to 4 minutes.

3. Remove from the heat and add the spinach. Stir in the cilantro and lime juice. Taste and adjust the flavors as needed. Add a squirt of hot sauce, if desired.

4. Serve warm, topped with additional cilantro, scallion greens, and Thai basil, if using. The soup is best eaten on the day it is made.

VARIATION TIP: If you're not dealing with mouth sores and are looking to add more heat to this soup, you can substitute red curry paste for yellow curry paste and add some chopped jalapeño.

PER SERVING: Calories: 646; Total fat: 24g; Sodium: 345mg; Carbohydrates: 84g; Fiber: 6g; Protein: 25g

# Spring Green Soup

| SERVES: 4 to 6 | PREP TIME: 10 Minutes | COOK TIME: 20 Minutes |
|---|---|---|

SYMPTOMS: Fatigue / Trouble Swallowing / Taste Changes / Sore Mouth or Throat / Unintentional Weight Loss / Constipation

2 tablespoons extra-virgin olive oil

1 leek, white and light green parts only, thinly sliced

½ teaspoon sea salt, or more as needed

4 cups frozen peas, thawed, or 3½ pounds fresh peas, shelled

4 cups vegetable broth (such as Mineral-Rich Vegetable Broth, page 158)

2 cups tightly packed fresh baby spinach

¼ cup chopped fresh flat-leaf parsley

¼ cup chopped fresh mint

¼ cup chopped fresh chives

1 cup plain full-fat Greek yogurt

1 teaspoon lemon juice

VARIATION TIP: To make this recipe vegan and dairy-free, you can substitute the yogurt with coconut yogurt or a plant-based milk, like unsweetened cashew, almond, or coconut.

Fresh spring vegetables and herbs enliven this colorful soup, which is full of anticancer nutrients, antioxidants, minerals, and vitamins. The soup offers a balanced blend of fiber, protein, and healthy fat. Enjoy it warm or chilled.

1. In a Dutch oven or large, deep pot, heat the oil over medium heat. Add the leek and salt, cover, and cook until soft and tender, stirring occasionally, about 10 minutes. Add the peas, pour in the broth, and bring to a simmer. Cover and cook until the peas are tender but still bright green, 5 to 8 minutes for frozen peas, 20 to 25 minutes for fresh peas.

2. Stir in the spinach, parsley, mint, and chives and cook for about 1 minute, until the greens are wilted. Puree the soup with an immersion blender (or in a blender, working in batches). Stir in the yogurt and lemon juice and add more salt, if needed.

3. Serve warm, at room temperature, or chilled. Store leftovers in an airtight container in the refrigerator for up to 5 days or in the freezer for up to 3 months.

PER SERVING: Calories: 234; Total fat: 10g; Sodium: 287mg; Carbohydrates: 28g; Fiber: 8g; Protein: 11g

# Veggie Lover's Chicken Soup

SERVES: **4** | PREP TIME: **10 Minutes** | COOK TIME: **20 Minutes**

SYMPTOMS: Nausea / Fatigue / Anemia / Taste Changes / Diarrhea

2 tablespoons extra-virgin olive oil

1 pound boneless, skinless chicken breasts, cut into bite-size pieces

2 medium zucchini, diced

2 large shallots, finely chopped

1 teaspoon herbes de Provence

¼ teaspoon sea salt

4 ripe plum tomatoes, chopped

4 cups bone broth (such as Mineral-Rich Bone Broth, page 160, or Basic Chicken Bone Broth, page 162)

½ cup dry white wine or apple cider vinegar

¼ cup orzo, orecchiette, ditalini, or other tiny pasta

2 cups chopped fresh spinach

Fresh lemon juice

Grated Parmesan or Romano cheese (optional)

There is something inherently comforting about chicken noodle soup. This version provides a generous serving of protein along with immune-boosting, anticancer nutrients from the vegetables and the bone broth.

1. In a Dutch oven or large, deep pot, heat the oil over medium-high heat. Add the chicken and cook until browned all over and cooked through, 3 to 4 minutes. Transfer to a plate.

2. Add the zucchini, shallots, herbes de Provence, and salt to the pot. Cook, stirring often, until the veggies are slightly softened, about 3 minutes.

3. Add the tomatoes, broth, wine, and orzo. Increase the heat to high and bring to a boil. Reduce to low and simmer until the pasta is tender, about 10 minutes.

4. Stir in the spinach and chicken. Simmer for another 5 minutes.

5. Serve with a squeeze of lemon juice and some grated Parmesan, if using. Store leftovers in an airtight container in the refrigerator for up to 4 days or in the freezer for up to 4 months.

PER SERVING: Calories: 260; Total fat: 10g; Sodium: 193mg; Carbohydrates: 12g; Fiber: 3g; Protein: 28g

# Chicken Tortilla Soup

SERVES: 4 to 6 | PREP TIME: 10 Minutes | COOK TIME: 20 Minutes

SYMPTOMS: Fatigue / Anemia / Taste Changes / Constipation

2 tablespoons extra-virgin olive oil

1 small onion, chopped

3 garlic cloves, minced or pressed

4 cups bone broth (such as Mineral-Rich Bone Broth, page 160, or Basic Chicken Bone Broth, page 162)

1 (14.5-ounce) can diced tomatoes

1 pound boneless, skinless chicken breasts

¾ tablespoon ground cumin

½ tablespoon chili powder

½ teaspoon sea salt

2 medium carrots, thinly sliced

½ cup chopped fresh cilantro, plus more for garnish

Juice of 1 lime, plus more for serving

Tortilla chips

2 avocados, pitted, peeled and diced

Shredded cheddar or Monterey Jack cheese (optional)

One of the things I miss the most since leaving California is its Mexican food, but this easy and tasty soup helps fill that craving. It's flavorful and zesty, yet comforting and light enough to be enjoyed in winter or summer. The vegetables and spices provide protein, healthy fat, antioxidants, and anticancer nutrients. I love that you can cook the whole chicken breasts right in the soup, which saves on initial prep time. To make it even easier, you can use leftover or rotisserie chicken from the store. Just add it at the end to warm it in the liquid.

1. In a Dutch oven or large, deep pot, heat the oil over medium-high heat. Add the onion and garlic and sauté until softened, about 3 minutes. Add the broth, tomatoes with their juice, chicken, cumin, chili powder, and salt. Submerge the chicken in the liquid, increase the heat to high, and bring to a boil. Add the carrots. Return to a boil, then reduce the heat to medium and cook for another 10 to 12 minutes, until the carrots are tender.

2. Using tongs, carefully remove the chicken from the pot and either shred or chop it. Put the chicken back in the pot and stir in the cilantro and lime juice.

3. Ladle the soup into bowls and serve topped with a handful of tortilla chips, avocado, more cilantro, cheese (if using), and a spritz more lime juice. Store any leftovers, without the toppings, in an airtight container in the refrigerator for up to 1 week or in the freezer for up to 4 months.

VARIATION TIP: Make it vegetarian by replacing the poultry with 1 (15-ounce) can of black beans and 1 cup of corn, and using Mineral-Rich Vegetable Broth (page 158) in place of bone broth.

PER SERVING: Calories: 428; Total fat: 26g; Sodium: 387mg; Carbohydrates: 23g; Fiber: 12g; Protein: 31g

# Lemony Chicken Soup

SERVES: **5** | PREP TIME: **10 Minutes** | COOK TiME: **20 Minutes**

SYMPTOMS: Nausea / Fatigue / Anemia / Taste Changes / Constipation

2 tablespoons extra-virgin olive oil

1 medium onion, quartered and thinly sliced

4 garlic cloves, minced or pressed

10 cups bone broth (such as Mineral-Rich Bone Broth, page 160, or Basic Chicken Bone Broth, page 162)

1 pound boneless, skinless chicken breasts

Grated zest and juice of 1 large lemon

½ teaspoon red pepper flakes

1 cup Israeli couscous

1 teaspoon sea salt, or more as needed

½ teaspoon freshly ground black pepper, or more as needed

½ cup crumbled feta cheese (about 3 ounces)

⅓ cup chopped fresh chives

A Mediterranean-inspired riff on a comfort food favorite, this chicken soup provides nourishment and is a good way to help meet your hydration needs. Lemon is a great addition for soothing nausea and helping with taste changes. This soup offers protein, iron, vitamin $B_{12}$, and vitamin C, plus anticancer and immune-boosting phytonutrients.

1. In a large Dutch oven or large, deep pot, heat the oil over medium-high heat. Add the onion and garlic and sauté for 3 to 4 minutes to soften. Add the broth, chicken, lemon zest and juice, and red pepper flakes. Increase the heat to high, cover, and bring to a boil. Once boiling, reduce the heat to medium and simmer, uncovered, for 10 minutes.

2. Stir in the couscous, salt, and pepper. Simmer for another 5 minutes to cook the couscous, then turn off the heat.

3. Using tongs, carefully remove the chicken from the pot and either shred or chop it. Put the chicken back in the pot, stir in the feta and chives, then taste and add more salt or pepper, if desired.

4. Serve. Store leftovers in an airtight container in the refrigerator for up to 1 week or in the freezer for up to 4 months.

VARIATION TIPS: You can omit the feta if you are dairy-free or substitute cooked quinoa or brown rice for the couscous if you are gluten-free. If you don't have 10 cups of broth on hand, you can use 5 cups broth and 5 cups water.

PER SERVING: Calories: 346; Total fat: 12g; Sodium: 551mg; Carbohydrates: 31g; Fiber: 2g; Protein: 28g

# Harira-Inspired Stew

| SERVES: 8 | PREP TIME: 10 Minutes | COOK TIME: 2 Hours |
| --- | --- | --- |

SYMPTOMS: Fatigue / Trouble Swallowing / Anemia / Taste Changes / Diarrhea

Drawing inspiration from harira, a traditional Moroccan soup that is often served during Ramadan, this is one of my favorite one-pot meals. This stew provides plenty of protein and fiber along with iron, vitamin C, and potassium. The long simmer time ensures a rich, flavorful soup, yet it's simple to pull together and can feed a crowd.

2 tablespoons extra-virgin olive oil

1 teaspoon ground turmeric

1 teaspoon ground ginger

1 teaspoon ground cinnamon

1 teaspoon sea salt

½ teaspoon freshly ground black pepper

Large pinch saffron

3 celery stalks, finely chopped (about 1 cup)

2 medium onions, finely chopped

6 garlic cloves, minced or pressed

1 cup chopped fresh flat-leaf parsley

1 pound boneless, skinless chicken thighs, cut into bite-size cubes

1 (28-ounce) can diced tomatoes

1½ cups cooked chickpeas, or 1 (15-ounce) can chickpeas, rinsed and drained

¾ cup green or brown lentils, rinsed

4 cups bone broth (such as Mineral-Rich Bone Broth, page 160, or Basic Chicken Bone Broth, page 162)

4 cups water

Lemon, cut into quarters

1. In a Dutch oven or large, deep pot, heat the olive oil over medium heat. Add the turmeric, ginger, cinnamon, salt, pepper, saffron, celery, onions, garlic, and parsley. Cook, stirring occasionally, until the vegetables soften, about 10 minutes.

2. Add the chicken and stir to combine. Continue to cook for another 10 minutes.

3. Add the tomatoes with their juice, chickpeas, lentils, broth, and water. Increase the heat to high and bring to a boil. Reduce the heat to low, cover, and simmer until the flavors are melded, about 90 minutes.

4. Serve the stew warm with a squeeze of fresh lemon juice. Store leftovers in an airtight container in the refrigerator for up to 1 week or in the freezer for up to 4 months.

VARIATION TIP: Feel free to omit the chicken for a vegan stew that is already a good source of protein, thanks to the chickpeas and lentils.

PER SERVING: Calories: 266; Total fat: 8g; Sodium: 421mg; Carbohydrates: 30g; Fiber: 8g; Protein: 21g

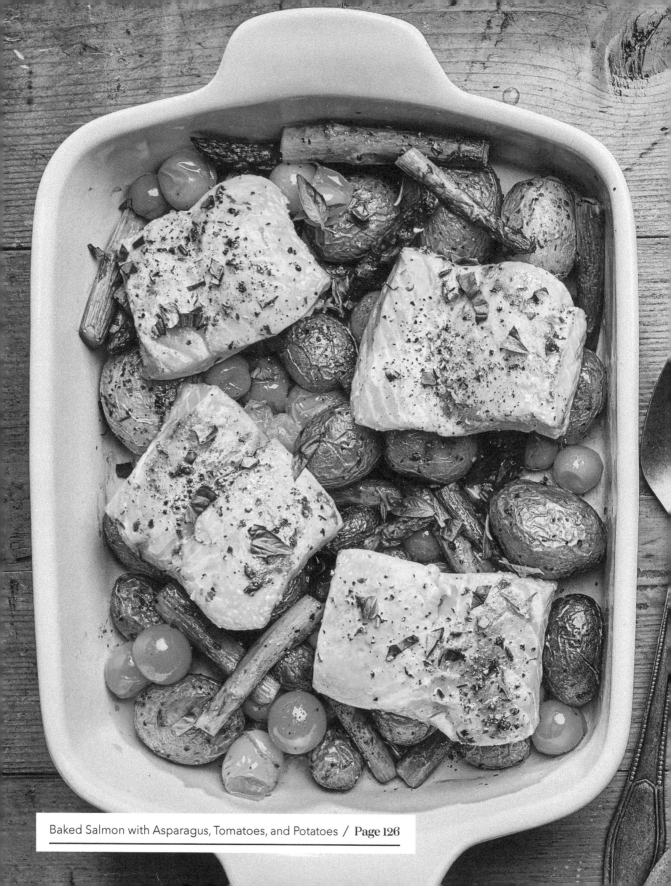

Baked Salmon with Asparagus, Tomatoes, and Potatoes / **Page 126**

# CHAPTER 6

# Strengthening Meals

# Spaghetti with Mushroom Bolognese

**SERVES: 6 to 8** | **PREP TIME: 10 Minutes** | **COOK TIME: 20 Minutes**

SYMPTOMS: Nausea / Fatigue / Anemia / Constipation

3 tablespoons unsalted butter (preferably grass-fed)

2 pounds fresh cremini mushrooms, trimmed and chopped

½ ounce dried porcini mushrooms, rinsed and minced

1 medium carrot, finely chopped

1 small onion, finely chopped

3 garlic cloves, minced or pressed

2 tablespoons tomato paste

1 (28-ounce) can diced tomatoes

1 tablespoon soy sauce

1 teaspoon dried oregano

½ teaspoon sea salt, or more as needed

¼ teaspoon freshly ground black pepper, or more as needed

¼ cup crème fraîche or heavy cream

1 (16-ounce) box whole-grain or gluten-free pasta (such as spaghetti or linguini)

Grated Parmesan cheese (optional)

A warm bowl of pasta is one of the ultimate comfort foods, and there's no reason it can't be included in your cancer-healing diet. By adding nourishing anticancer foods, like mushrooms, onions, garlic, and tomatoes, you can easily transform this dish into a healing meal.

1. In a Dutch oven or large, deep pot, melt the butter over medium heat. Add the cremini and porcini mushrooms, carrot, and onion and cook until the vegetables soften and begin to brown, 12 to 15 minutes.

2. Stir in the garlic and cook until fragrant, about 30 seconds. Stir in the tomato paste and cook for another minute. Add the tomatoes with their juice, soy sauce, oregano, salt, and pepper. Stir together and bring to a simmer. Reduce the heat to medium-low and simmer until the sauce has thickened a bit, 8 to 10 minutes. Remove from the heat and stir in the crème fraîche.

3. Meanwhile, in a large pot, cook the pasta according to the package instructions, reserving some of the cooking water.

4. Drain and add the pasta to the sauce. Toss to combine, adding some of the reserved cooking water as needed to achieve a creamy consistency. Add more salt or pepper if needed.

5. Serve the pasta warm with Parmesan sprinkled on top, if using. Store leftovers in an airtight container in the refrigerator for up to 5 days or in the freezer for up to 2 months.

VARIATION TIPS: To make this meal dairy-free, use extra-virgin olive oil instead of butter and either omit the cream or use a plant-based option. To make the meal gluten-free, use a gluten-free soy sauce and gluten-free noodles.

PER SERVING: Calories: 462; Total fat: 12g; Sodium: 526mg; Carbohydrates: 77g; Fiber: 10g; Protein: 16g

# Black Bean–Stuffed Sweet Potatoes

| SERVES: 4 | PREP: 5 Minutes | COOK: 1 Hour 15 Minutes |

SYMPTOMS: Nausea / Fatigue / Trouble Swallowing / Anemia / Taste Changes / Diarrhea / Constipation

4 medium sweet potatoes

1½ tablespoons extra-virgin olive oil

1 small red onion, finely chopped

½ teaspoon ground cumin

½ teaspoon chili powder

½ teaspoon sea salt

1 (15-ounce) can black beans, rinsed and drained

2 avocados, pitted, peeled, and diced

Chopped fresh cilantro

Juice of 1 lime

Sour cream or crème fraîche (optional)

Sweet potatoes are one of my absolute favorite vegetables. These root vegetables are not only delicious but also loaded with anti-inflammatory, anticancer nutrients. Black beans are also an excellent source of fiber, in addition to providing protein, iron, and B vitamins. The avocado offers healthy fat, while the spices and cilantro give this meal an extra tasty (and anticancer) kick.

1. Preheat the oven to 350°F.

2. Wrap the sweet potatoes individually in foil and bake until tender, about 1 hour.

3. In a medium pan, heat the olive oil over medium heat. Add the onion and cook until translucent, about 5 minutes. Add the cumin, chili powder, and salt and cook for another 3 minutes. Add the black beans and cook, stirring frequently, until heated through, about 5 minutes more. Remove from the heat.

4.  Slice the warm sweet potatoes down the middle lengthwise and scoop out the insides to make "bowls." Divide the black bean mixture among the 8 potato halves. Top each with some diced avocado, fresh cilantro, a squeeze of lime juice, and sour cream, if using. Serve immediately, offering 2 stuffed halves per person.

PREP AHEAD TIP: You can bake the sweet potatoes and make the black bean mixture ahead of time. Follow the directions through step 4 and then let everything cool. Store separately in airtight containers in the refrigerator for up to 5 days. When ready to eat, reheat the potatoes and beans either on the stovetop or in the microwave and then fill the potatoes. To make this a vegan dish, simply omit the sour cream.

PER SERVING: Calories: 468; Total fat: 21g; Sodium: 321mg; Carbohydrates: 63g; Fiber: 21g; Protein: 13g

# Tofu and Mushroom Stir-Fry with Bok Choy

| SERVES: 4 | PREP TIME: 20 Minutes | COOK TIME: 15 Minutes |

SYMPTOMS: Fatigue / Anemia / Taste Changes / Constipation

1 (12-ounce) block extra-firm organic tofu

2 tablespoons avocado oil or other high-smoke-point oil

2 tablespoons soy sauce, divided

2 cups sliced fresh shiitake mushrooms

1 large or 3 baby bok choy, roughly chopped

5 scallions, white parts only, thinly sliced (about ½ cup)

4 garlic cloves, minced or pressed

½ cup vegetable broth (such as Mineral-Rich Vegetable Broth, page 158)

1 tablespoon minced fresh ginger

1 tablespoon cold-pressed organic toasted sesame oil

2 tablespoons sesame seeds

Cooked rice, quinoa, or noodles, warmed

A stir-fry is a simple, quick, and tasty way to add more vegetables and cancer-healing foods to your diet. Packed full of leafy greens, mushrooms, and tofu, this stir-fry supports good digestion, hormone balance, and a strong immune system. If you are gluten-free, choose a gluten-free soy sauce.

1. Wrap the tofu in a dish towel and place a plate on top. Let it sit for 10 to 15 minutes. Remove the plate, unwrap the tofu, and cut into ½-inch cubes.

2. In a large pan or wok, heat the avocado oil and 1 tablespoon of the soy sauce over medium-high heat. Add the tofu and fry, stirring occasionally, until all sides are lightly brown, 5 to 7 minutes. Transfer the tofu to a plate.

3. Reduce the heat to medium, then add the mushrooms and sauté for about 5 minutes, until tender. Add the remaining 1 tablespoon of soy sauce, bok choy, scallions, and garlic. Cook 1 to 2 minutes more. Reduce the heat to low and add the broth and ginger. Stir to combine and simmer until heated through and fragrant, another 2 to 3 minutes.

4. Return the tofu to the pan, stir in the sesame oil and sesame seeds, and toss together.

5. Serve the stir-fry over rice, quinoa, or noodles. Store leftovers in an airtight container in the refrigerator for up to 5 days or in the freezer for up to 3 weeks.

FLAVOR BOOST TIP: Feel free to adjust the flavors of this stir-fry to your liking. Add a tablespoon of honey for sweetness or to cut any metallic or bitter tastes you may be experiencing. You can add 2 to 4 tablespoons of lime juice for acidity, or a teaspoon of sriracha or other hot sauce to add heat.

PER SERVING: Calories: 218; Total fat: 18g; Sodium: 398mg; Carbohydrates: 6g; Fiber: 2g; Protein: 11g

# Veggie Frittata

**5**

**30**

**OP**

**VG**

| SERVES: 4 to 6 | PREP TIME: 5 Minutes | COOK TIME: 25 Minutes |
|---|---|---|

SYMPTOMS: Fatigue / Trouble Swallowing / Anemia / Constipation

2 tablespoons extra-virgin
  olive oil

1 leek, light green and white
  parts only, thinly sliced

4 cups fresh baby spinach

8 large eggs

2 teaspoons ground cumin

½ teaspoon sea salt

¼ teaspoon freshly ground
  black pepper

½ cup crumbled feta
  (about 2 ounces; optional)

VARIATION TIP: You can
easily substitute the kale or
chard for spinach, or use other
leafy greens.

A frittata is a baked Italian egg dish that's a lot
like a crustless quiche, which makes it a great
option for people who are avoiding grains. Eggs
are a great source of protein, as well as iron,
vitamin D, antioxidants, and healthy fats. This
recipe lends itself to the addition of any number
of vegetables, herbs, or spices. If you don't have
an oven-safe skillet, you can bake the frittata in
a lightly greased 9-by-13-inch baking dish.

1. Preheat the oven to 375°F.

2. In an oven-safe skillet, such as cast iron, heat the
   oil over medium heat. Add the leek and sauté until
   soft, 2 to 3 minutes. Add the spinach and cook until
   it just starts to wilt, about 1 minute more.

3. In a medium bowl, whisk the eggs with the cumin,
   salt, pepper, and feta, if using.

4. Pour the egg mixture over the vegetables and
   bake until the eggs are just set, 20 to 25 minutes.
   (Alternatively, if you're using a baking dish, spread
   the sautéed vegetables in an even layer, pour the
   egg mixture on top, and bake.)

5. Serve warm. Store leftovers in an airtight container in the refrigerator for up to 5 days or in the
   freezer for up to 3 months.

PER SERVING: Calories: 227; Total fat: 17g; Sodium: 405mg; Carbohydrates: 5g; Fiber: 1g; Protein: 14g

# Mushroom Burgers

| SERVES: 4 | PREP TIME: 5 Minutes | COOK TIME: 10 Minutes |

SYMPTOMS: Fatigue / Anemia / Diarrhea / Constipation

Mushrooms are one of my favorite cancer-healing foods because they support the immune system, improve digestion, lower inflammation, and balance hormones. They're also on the short list of foods that contain vitamin D. There is no end to the variety of toppings and veggies you can serve with these "burgers." This recipe uses the stovetop, but I also love these cooked on the grill, about 4 minutes per side over direct heat. Serve with Kale Salad (page 74) and Roasted Sweet Potato Fries (page 68) for a delicious and nourishing anticancer meal.

1 garlic clove, peeled
½ teaspoon sea salt
2 tablespoons plus
  1 teaspoon extra-virgin
  olive oil

4 portobello mushrooms,
  stems removed
4 whole-grain or
  gluten-free buns, cut in
  half and toasted

OPTIONAL TOPPINGS
Tomato slices, sliced avocado, sprouts, salad greens,
  Healthy Homemade
  Mayonnaise (page 176),
  and Basil-Spinach Pesto
  (page 172)

1. On a cutting board, mash the garlic and salt together with the flat side of a knife until it's a smooth paste. Transfer the paste to a small dish and mix with 2 tablespoons of the olive oil. Brush the mixture over the mushrooms.

2. Heat the remaining 1 teaspoon of oil in a large skillet over medium heat. Place the mushroom caps in the pan, top side down. Cook until browned and softened, about 5 minutes, then flip the mushrooms and cook until softened and golden brown, about 3 minutes more.

3. Build your mushroom burger on the buns with an assortment of toppings and serve immediately.

PER SERVING: Calories: 196; Total fat: 9g; Sodium: 390mg; Carbohydrates: 25g; Fiber: 2g; Protein: 6g

# Baked Salmon with Asparagus, Tomatoes, and Potatoes

| SERVES: 4 | PREP TIME: 5 Minutes | COOK TIME: 1 Hour |
|---|---|---|

SYMPTOMS: Fatigue / Anemia / Unintentional Weight Loss

1 pound baby potatoes

3 tablespoons extra-virgin olive oil, divided

1 teaspoon herbes de Provence, divided

½ teaspoon sea salt, divided

¼ teaspoon freshly ground black pepper, divided

1 small bunch fresh asparagus (about 8 ounces), trimmed and cut in half

1 pint cherry tomatoes

4 (4-ounce) wild-caught salmon fillets

2 tablespoons balsamic vinegar

½ cup chopped fresh basil

Wild-caught salmon is an excellent source of omega-3 fatty acids, plus antioxidants, vitamin $B_{12}$, zinc, and iron. It pairs really well with asparagus, tomatoes, and potatoes in this preparation. The asparagus is a great source of fiber, along with many different vitamins and minerals, while the tomatoes provide a good dose of vitamin C and other antioxidants. Although this recipe takes an hour from start to finish, the steps are simple and the result is reliably delicious.

1. Preheat the oven to 400°F.

2. In a 9-by-13-inch baking dish, toss the potatoes with 1 tablespoon of the olive oil, ½ teaspoon of the herbes de Provence, ¼ teaspoon of the salt, and ⅛ teaspoon of the pepper. Cover the dish with aluminum foil and roast until the potatoes start to soften, about 30 minutes.

3.  Add the asparagus to the pan, toss the vegetables to coat with the oil, and bake, uncovered, until the potatoes start to brown and the asparagus softens, about 15 minutes.

4.  Add the tomatoes to the pan, and nestle the salmon in the vegetables. Sprinkle with the remaining 2 tablespoons of oil, remaining ½ teaspoon of herbes de Provence, remaining ¼ teaspoon of salt, remaining ⅛ teaspoon of pepper, and the vinegar. Return to the oven to bake for 10 minutes, or until the salmon is just cooked through and starting to flake, and with a little translucency still in the thickest part.

5.  Sprinkle the basil leaves over the top and serve.

VARIATION TIP: If you don't have herbes de Provence or can't find the mix at your store, don't worry. You can use any dried herbs you do have; an Italian blend would work well or use individual herbs like rosemary, oregano, or thyme. Fennel seed in particular pairs well with fish.

PER SERVING: Calories: 370; Total fat: 18g; Sodium: 296mg; Carbohydrates: 26g; Fiber: 5g; Protein: 27g

# Easy Lemon-Butter Fish

| SERVES: 4 | PREP TIME: 5 Minutes | COOK TIME: 10 Minutes |

SYMPTOMS: Nausea / Fatigue / Trouble Swallowing / Anemia

One of the healthiest things you can do for your diet is eat more fish. Fish is an excellent source of protein, minerals, and omega-3 fatty acids. Omega-3s help the body heal from cancer, keep inflammation down, and support the immune system. This is one of the easiest and quickest ways to prepare fish. I've used this recipe with many different types of fish, including halibut, cod, trout, salmon, and arctic char, and it has always turned out delicious. Serve with side dishes such as Golden Cauliflower (page 69) and Kale Salad (page 74).

1 teaspoon extra-virgin olive oil

4 (4-ounce) skinless halibut or cod fillets

1 tablespoon unsalted butter (preferably grass-fed), cut into 8 pats

2 lemons, 1 sliced and 1 cut into wedges

½ teaspoon herbes de Provence

¼ teaspoon sea salt

1. In a large pan, heat the olive oil over medium heat. Place the fish fillets in the pan with 2 pats of butter and 2 or 3 lemon slices on top of each one. Sprinkle each fillet with the herbes de Provence, salt, and a squeeze of fresh lemon juice.

2. Cook, uncovered, for about 5 minutes. Carefully flip the fish and cook on the other side until the fish is just cooked through, another 5 minutes, depending on the thickness (10 minutes cooking per 1 inch of thickness). Fish cooks quickly, so be careful not to dry it out.

3. Serve immediately, squeezing more lemon over the fillets.

INGREDIENT TIP: Although all fish and shellfish contain omega-3 fatty acids, some are a richer source than others. To get the maximum amount of omega-3s, choose wild-caught cold-water fish like salmon and halibut.

PER SERVING: Calories: 141; Total fat: 5g; Sodium: 223mg; Carbohydrates: 1g; Fiber: 0g; Protein: 21g

# Tuna Pesto Pasta with Broccoli

SERVES: 6 | PREP TIME: 5 Minutes | COOK TIME: 15 Minutes

SYMPTOMS: Fatigue / Anemia / Unintentional Weight Loss / Constipation

This is a quick and easy meal that's well balanced with protein, healthy fat, and fiber. Canned tuna is an excellent protein source to keep in the pantry and is easy to use as a supplement to a dish when you need more protein. Wild-caught tuna provides more omega-3 fatty acids, while light tuna has been shown to be lower in mercury than albacore. Feel free to use a store-bought pesto to help save time.

Salt

1 (16-ounce) box whole-grain or gluten-free pasta (such as penne, shells, or rotini)

2 tablespoons extra-virgin olive oil

2 cups finely chopped broccoli florets

2 (5-ounce) cans wild-caught water-packed light tuna, drained

½ cup pesto (such as Basil-Spinach Pesto, page 172)

3 garlic cloves, minced or pressed

Freshly grated Parmesan cheese (optional)

1. Bring a large pot of water and a pinch of salt to a boil. Add the pasta and cook according to the package instructions. Drain the pasta, reserving some pasta water, and return it to the pot.

2. While the pasta is cooking, heat the olive oil in a large skillet over medium-low heat. Add the broccoli, tuna, pesto, and garlic and stir to combine. Cover and cook over low heat until the broccoli is tender and the other ingredients are heated through, about 10 minutes.

3. Add the tuna mixture to the pasta and toss to combine, adding a little pasta cooking water as needed to lighten the consistency.

4. Serve the pasta warm, topped with a sprinkling of Parmesan, if using. Store leftovers in an airtight container in the refrigerator for up to 3 days.

PER SERVING: Calories: 485; Total fat: 19g; Sodium: 160mg; Carbohydrates: 59g; Fiber: 3g; Protein: 19g

# Herb-Roasted Chicken and Potatoes

| SERVES: 6 | PREP: 10 Minutes | COOK: 1 Hour 30 Minutes |

SYMPTOMS: Fatigue / Anemia / Unintentional Weight Loss

3 to 6 sprigs assorted fresh herbs (such as rosemary, thyme, and sage)

2 dried bay leaves

2 pounds fingerling potatoes, halved or quartered (depending on their size)

2 large shallots, chopped

7 garlic cloves, 4 minced and 3 left whole

2 tablespoons extra-virgin olive oil, divided

½ teaspoon sea salt, divided

½ teaspoon freshly ground black pepper, divided

2 tablespoons herbes de Provence, divided

1 (4-pound) roasting chicken (preferably organic and pasture-raised)

1 tablespoon fennel seeds

One of the most nourishing and comforting meals that we enjoy in my family is roast chicken. It takes some time to cook, but it is easy and quick to prepare, and it's always a crowd-pleaser. The shallots, garlic, and herbs are great immune-boosting, anticancer additions. The fennel seeds add a distinct and delicious flavor, and also help support digestion. What's even more wonderful about this meal is that when you're finished eating it, you can make a nourishing and healing bone broth with the chicken carcass (see pages 160 and 162).

1. Preheat the oven to 400°F.

2. Tie the fresh herbs and bay leaves together in a bundle using butcher's twine.

3. In a large Dutch oven or a large roasting pan, combine the potatoes, shallots, and the 4 minced garlic cloves. Add 1 tablespoon of the olive oil, ¼ teaspoon of the salt, ¼ teaspoon of the pepper, and 1 tablespoon of the herbes de Provence. Mix well until everything is coated; I like to use my hands for this.

4.  Make a space in the middle of the potatoes and place the chicken, breast side up. Insert the 3 whole garlic cloves and the bundle of herbs in the chicken cavity. Rub the outside of the chicken with the remaining 1 tablespoon of olive oil, remaining ¼ teaspoon of salt, remaining ¼ teaspoon of pepper, and remaining 1 tablespoon of herbes de Provence. Sprinkle the fennel seeds over everything in the pan.

5.  Cover with a lid or aluminum foil and roast until the chicken and potatoes are tender and golden, about 90 minutes. Uncover the chicken for the last 15 to 20 minutes to let the skin brown. The chicken is done when the thickest part of the thigh has reached an internal temperature of 165°F.

6.  Let the chicken rest for about 10 minutes to redistribute the juices through the meat. Carve the chicken by first separating the legs and wings from the body, then the thighs from the drumsticks, and then finally the 2 sides of the breast from the center breastbone.

7.  Transfer the chicken to a platter, add the roasted potatoes, and serve. Store leftovers in an airtight container in the refrigerator for up to 4 days.

PER SERVING: Calories: 480; Total fat: 28g; Sodium: 262mg; Carbohydrates: 28g; Fiber: 4g; Protein: 29g

# Turkey-Stuffed Zucchini

| SERVES: 4 to 6 | PREP TIME: 5 Minutes | COOK TIME: 30 Minutes |

SYMPTOMS: Nausea / Fatigue / Anemia / Constipation

2 tablespoons extra-virgin olive oil, divided

2 shallots, chopped

1 pound ground turkey

8 ounces fresh cremini mushrooms, chopped

1 tablespoon herbes de Provence

½ teaspoon sea salt

¼ teaspoon freshly ground black pepper

6 medium zucchini (about 2 pounds)

2 ripe large heirloom tomatoes, chopped (optional)

Freshly grated Parmesan cheese (optional)

Zucchini is a summer staple in my house. I'm always looking for new ways to cook with it, and this one was a hit. Zucchini is rich in several different vitamins and minerals, most notably vitamin C, vitamin A, manganese, potassium, and magnesium. The shallots, mushrooms, and tomatoes further boost the cancer-healing benefits of this dish, and the ground turkey provides a great dose of protein, iron, and minerals. Serve with a side salad.

1. Preheat the oven to 400°F. Line a baking sheet with parchment.

2. In a large skillet, heat 1 tablespoon of the olive oil over medium heat. Add the shallots and sauté until soft and transparent, 2 to 3 minutes. Add the ground turkey, mushrooms, herbes de Provence, salt, and pepper. Stir together and break up the turkey into smaller bits. Cook until the turkey is browned and the mushrooms are soft, 5 to 8 minutes.

3. Cut the zucchini in half lengthwise and scoop the seeds and some of the soft flesh out of the middle of each, creating a space for the turkey mixture. Place on the baking sheet and drizzle the remaining 1 tablespoon of olive oil over the zucchini, rubbing it into the flesh.

4. Fill the middle of each zucchini boat with the turkey mixture. Top with the chopped tomatoes and cheese, if using. Bake for about 20 minutes, until the zucchini is soft and the tops are browned.

5. Serve warm. Store leftovers in an airtight container in the refrigerator for up to 4 days or in the freezer for up to 6 months.

PER SERVING: Calories: 291; Total fat: 17g; Sodium: 335mg; Carbohydrates: 11g; Fiber: 4g; Protein: 25g

# Moroccan-Spiced Chicken

SERVES: **6** | PREP: **20 Minutes** | COOK: **2 Hours 40 Minutes**

SYMPTOMS: Fatigue / Trouble Swallowing / Anemia / Taste Changes

2 teaspoons ground cumin

1½ teaspoons ground ginger

1½ teaspoons sea salt

1 teaspoon ground turmeric

1 teaspoon ground paprika

½ teaspoon ground cinnamon

½ teaspoon freshly ground
black pepper

3 tablespoons extra-virgin
olive oil, divided

4 garlic cloves, minced
or pressed

6 boneless, skinless
chicken thighs

1 large lemon (preferably
Meyer), cut into 8 wedges

4 large red
potatoes, quartered

1 large onion, chopped

8 dates (preferably Medjool),
pitted and halved

14 green olives, pitted

1 cup coarsely chopped fresh
flat-leaf parsley

1 cup bone broth (such as
Mineral-Rich Bone Broth,
page 160, or Basic Chicken
Bone Broth, page 162)

The spices in this crowd-pleasing chicken dish provide anti-inflammatory and immune-boosting benefits, making it an essential cancer-healing meal. Yes, it takes some time to cook, but the prep is easy and the long cook time results in a chicken that will melt in your mouth. Serve with cooked vegetables or a side salad.

1. In a medium bowl, mix the cumin, ginger, salt, turmeric, paprika, cinnamon, and pepper with 2 tablespoons of the olive oil and the garlic. Add the chicken and coat it with the mixture. Let the chicken sit for 15 minutes.

2. Meanwhile, in a Dutch oven or large, deep pot, heat the remaining 1 tablespoon of olive oil over medium heat. Add the chicken and brown on both sides, about 5 minutes per side.

3. Add the lemon, potatoes, onion, dates, olives, parsley, and broth. Stir together. Reduce the heat to low, cover, and simmer until the chicken is so tender it falls off the bone and the mixture smells aromatic, about 2½ hours.

4. Serve warm, with cooked vegetables or a side salad. Store leftovers in an airtight container in the refrigerator for up to 4 days.

PREP AHEAD TIP: This preparation also works well in a slow cooker. Some cookers even allow you to brown the chicken before adding the other ingredients. Simply prep everything in the morning, set the cooker on low, and then leave to cook all day or at least 8 hours.

PER SERVING: Calories: 493; Total fat: 13g; Sodium: 550mg; Carbohydrates: 69g; Fiber: 8g; Protein: 28g

# Turkey Taco Salad

**30**

| SERVES: 6 to 8 | PREP TIME: 10 Minutes | COOK TIME: 15 Minutes |
| --- | --- | --- |

SYMPTOMS: Fatigue / Anemia / Taste Changes

2 tablespoons extra-virgin olive oil

1 pound ground turkey

1 (1-ounce) packet organic taco seasoning

1 (15-ounce) can black beans, rinsed and drained

½ teaspoon ground cumin

1 (10-ounce) bag frozen yellow corn kernels, or 4 ears of corn, cooked and kernels cut off the cobs

1 head romaine lettuce, roughly chopped

1 medium cucumber, peeled and cubed

2 avocados, pitted, peeled, and diced

1 (13-ounce) bag organic tortilla chips

1 cup Fresh Salsa (page 175)

1 bunch fresh cilantro, coarsely chopped

½ cup Lime-Garlic Dressing (see variation, page 168)

Grated cheddar or Monterey Jack cheese (optional)

Sour cream (optional)

I like to serve this dish, which combines the best elements of both tacos and salads, on a hot summer day. This meal is packed with protein, fiber, iron, B vitamins, vitamin C, and immune-boosting anticancer phytonutrients. You can serve it as a main course or share it at your next potluck, barbecue, or picnic.

1. In a large skillet, heat the olive oil over medium heat. Add the turkey, breaking it up into pieces with a wooden spoon. Cook until it starts to brown, 6 to 8 minutes. Add the taco seasoning and stir to combine. Turn off the burner and cover to keep warm.

2. In a small saucepan, combine the beans with a splash of water and the cumin, then stir to combine. Heat through over low heat, about 5 minutes. Turn off the burner and cover to keep warm.

3. In a second small saucepan, heat the corn over low heat, about 5 minutes. Turn off the burner and cover to keep warm.

4. Divide the lettuce among 4 large bowls. Top each with some of the turkey, black beans, and corn, then add the cucumber and avocado. Crumble the chips over each salad and top with the salsa, cilantro, dressing, and cheese and sour cream, if using.

5. Serve immediately. Store leftovers of the ingredients in separate airtight containers in the refrigerator for up to 4 days.

VARIATION TIP: To make this meal vegan or vegetarian, simply omit the turkey and double the amount of beans and corn.

PER SERVING: Calories: 764; Total fat: 30g; Sodium: 143mg; Carbohydrates: 90g; Fiber: 21g; Protein: 43g

# Curried Chicken with Chickpeas

| SERVES: 6 | PREP TIME: 10 Minutes | COOK TIME: 40 Minutes |
|---|---|---|

SYMPTOMS: Fatigue / Trouble Swallowing / Anemia / Taste Changes / Constipation

2 tablespoons extra-virgin olive oil

2 large onions, chopped

2 teaspoons ground cumin

2 teaspoons ground coriander

2 teaspoons ground turmeric

2 teaspoons curry powder

½ teaspoon chili powder

½ teaspoon sea salt

¼ teaspoon freshly ground black pepper

4 garlic cloves, minced or pressed

1½ tablespoons minced fresh ginger (from 2-inch piece)

6 boneless, skinless chicken thighs or breasts, cut into bite-size pieces

2 cups bone broth (such as Mineral-Rich Bone Broth, page 160, or Basic Chicken Bone Broth, page 162)

1½ cups cooked chickpeas, or 1 (15-ounce) can chickpeas, rinsed and drained

Inspired by the flavors of India, this irresistible curry is a great source of protein, iron, B vitamins, vitamin C, and fiber. It also keeps well in both the refrigerator and the freezer, making it a good option to cook in advance and then pull out for a quick lunch or dinner.

1. In a Dutch oven or large, deep pot, heat the olive oil over medium heat. Add the onions and sauté until soft and translucent, 6 to 8 minutes. Add the cumin, coriander, turmeric, curry powder, chili powder, salt, pepper, garlic, and ginger, stirring constantly to prevent the spices from sticking. Cook until fragrant, about 2 minutes.

2. Add the chicken, broth, chickpeas, and tomatoes with their juice. Stir, reduce the heat to low, cover, and simmer for about 30 minutes, until the chicken is cooked through and fork-tender.

3. Add the greens and cook just until wilted, about 2 minutes more.

1 (15-ounce) can
    diced tomatoes
3 cups fresh greens (such as
    baby spinach, baby kale, or
    young chard)
Cooked rice or other
    grain, warmed

4. Serve warm, with a side of rice or another grain.
   Store leftovers in an airtight container in the
   refrigerator for up to 7 days or in the freezer for
   up to 3 months.

VARIATION TIP: If you find the heat of the spices to be too
much, decrease the amounts, especially the ginger, garlic,
and chili powder. Or top each bowl with some chopped
fresh mint and a dollop of plain yogurt, which helps cool
the heat.

PER SERVING: Calories: 255; Total fat: 8g; Sodium: 413mg; Carbohydrates: 19g; Fiber: 6g; Protein: 27g

# Turkey and Bean Chili

| SERVES: 8 | PREP TIME: 5 Minutes | COOK TIME: 2 Hours |
|---|---|---|

SYMPTOMS: Fatigue / Trouble Swallowing / Anemia / Taste Changes / Unintentional Weight Loss / Constipation

There are many great chili recipes out there, but this one is my family's favorite. It's warm, comforting, flavorful, and filling, while also being a great source of protein, fiber, antioxidants, and immune-boosting, anti-inflammatory, anticancer spices. You can easily make this a vegan meal by omitting the turkey, or increase the iron content by substituting organic grass-fed ground beef for the turkey.

2 tablespoons extra-virgin olive oil

2 medium onions, chopped

1 red bell pepper, cored, seeded, and chopped

6 garlic cloves, minced or pressed

¼ cup chili powder

1 tablespoon ground cumin

2 teaspoons ground coriander

1 teaspoon dried oregano

½ teaspoon red pepper flakes

2 pounds ground turkey

1 (28-ounce) can dark red kidney beans, rinsed and drained

1 (28-ounce) can diced tomatoes

1 (28-ounce) can crushed tomatoes

2 cups bone broth (such as Mineral-Rich Bone Broth, page 160, or Basic Chicken Bone Broth, page 162)

1 teaspoon sea salt, or more as needed

Cornbread or crusty whole-grain bread

Lime wedges

Maple syrup or honey (optional)

1. In a Dutch oven or large, deep pot, heat the olive oil over medium heat. Stir in the onions, bell pepper, garlic, chili powder, cumin, coriander, oregano, and red pepper flakes. Cook, stirring occasionally, until the vegetables start to soften, about 10 minutes.

2. Increase the heat to medium-high and add the turkey, breaking it up with a wooden spoon. Cook until it starts to brown, 6 to 8 minutes.

3. Add the beans, tomatoes with their juice, broth, and salt and let it come to a boil. Reduce the heat to low and simmer, partially covered, until the turkey is tender and the chili is dark and slightly thickened, about 90 minutes. Taste and add salt, if needed.

4. Serve warm with a side of warm cornbread or crusty bread. Spritz the top with lime juice and drizzle on some maple syrup or honey, if needed, to balance the spice. Store leftovers in an airtight container in the refrigerator for up to 4 days or in the freezer for up to 6 months.

PER SERVING: Calories: 378; Total fat: 15g; Sodium: 389mg; Carbohydrates: 34g; Fiber: 13g; Protein: 32g

# Walnut Chicken with Pomegranate

| SERVES: 6 | PREP: 10 Minutes | COOK: 1 Hour 40 Minutes |

SYMPTOMS: Fatigue / Trouble Swallowing / Anemia / Taste Changes / Unintentional Weight Loss / Constipation

2 tablespoons unsalted butter (preferably grass-fed), divided

3 tablespoons extra-virgin olive oil, divided

2 pounds boneless, skinless chicken thighs, cut into 1-inch strips

½ teaspoon sea salt

2 medium onions, chopped

2 cups bone broth (such as Mineral-Rich Bone Broth, page 160, or Basic Chicken Bone Broth, page 162)

2 cups raw walnut halves (about 8 ounces), toasted

1 teaspoon ground turmeric

½ teaspoon ground cinnamon

½ teaspoon ground nutmeg

¼ teaspoon freshly ground black pepper

1 cup pomegranate seeds

Cooked rice, warmed

Another family favorite at my house is this delicious chicken stew, inspired by a popular Iranian dish called fesenjan. The toasted walnuts add such fantastic flavor, in addition to healthy fat and antioxidants, and the pomegranate provides extra vitamin C, folate, and potassium. It takes a bit of time to make but is absolutely worth it. The leftovers are even better the next day, and it holds up well in the freezer.

1. In a large skillet, heat 1 tablespoon of the butter and 2 tablespoons of the olive oil over medium-high heat. When the butter is melted, place the chicken strips in the pan, sprinkle with the salt, and sauté until lightly browned, 3 to 4 minutes per side. Work in batches, if necessary, to avoid crowding. Transfer the chicken to a plate.

2. Add the remaining 1 tablespoon of butter and remaining 1 tablespoon of oil to the pan. Reduce the heat to medium-low, add the onions, and sauté until translucent, 8 to 10 minutes.

3. Return the chicken to the pan and add the broth. Increase the heat to high and bring to a boil. Reduce the heat to low, cover, and simmer until the chicken is tender and cooked through, about 30 minutes.

4. Meanwhile, pulse the walnuts in a food processor until finely ground.

5. Stir the walnuts, turmeric, cinnamon, nutmeg, and pepper into the chicken mixture. Cover and cook until the sauce is darkened and slightly thickened, stirring occasionally to prevent the walnuts from sticking to the pan, about 1 hour.

6. Serve over rice and top with the pomegranate seeds. Store leftovers in an airtight container in the refrigerator for up to 4 days or in the freezer for up to 6 months.

VARIATION TIP: To make this recipe dairy-free, simply substitute additional olive oil for the butter.

PER SERVING: Calories: 535; Total fat: 37g; Sodium: 227mg; Carbohydrates: 14g; Fiber: 4g; Protein: 40g

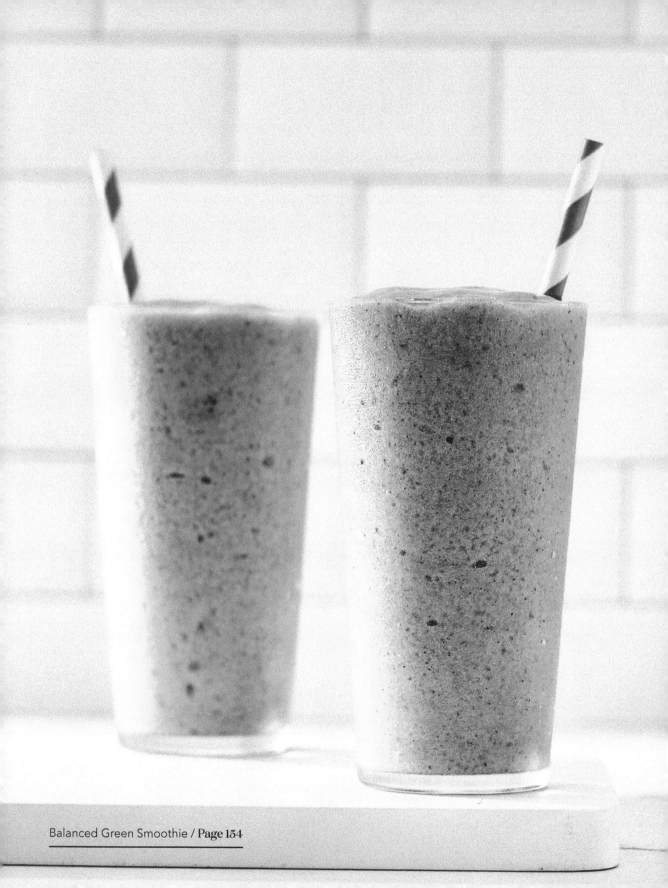

Balanced Green Smoothie / **Page 154**

CHAPTER 7

# Drinks and Tonics

# Morning Tonic

| SERVES: 2 | PREP TIME: 5 Minutes | COOK TIME: 3 Minutes |

SYMPTOMS: Nausea / Taste Changes / Diarrhea / Constipation

1 tablespoon grated fresh turmeric (from 2-inch piece)

1 tablespoon grated fresh ginger (from 2-inch piece)

Grated zest and juice of 1 lemon

4 cups filtered water, or more as needed

1 to 2 teaspoons maple syrup or raw honey (optional)

I love to drink this healing tonic first thing in the morning, before starting my day or eating anything. This drink warms and hydrates you, boosts detoxification, and prepares the gut for digestion. It also soothes nausea and stomach upset, while also offering anti-inflammatory and immune-boosting benefits.

1.  In a small saucepan, stir together the turmeric, ginger, lemon zest and juice, and water and bring to a simmer over medium heat, about 3 minutes.

2.  Taste and add 1 to 2 teaspoons of maple syrup, depending on how sweet you like it. If it's too strong, dilute with more water.

3.  Strain into 2 mugs and serve.

PREP AHEAD TIP: If you want to make sure you have this tonic at the ready without having to make it each morning, simply double or triple the recipe and store it in an airtight container in the refrigerator for up to 3 days. Reheat it on the stovetop or in the microwave until just warm.

PER SERVING: Calories: 12; Total fat: 0g; Sodium: 1mg; Carbohydrates: 3g; Fiber: 1g; Protein: 0g

# Soothing Throat Elixir

5
OP
V

| SERVES: 2 | PREP TIME: 5 Minutes, plus 12 hours to sit | COOK TIME: 15 Minutes |
|---|---|---|

SYMPTOMS: Nausea / Taste Changes / Sore Mouth or Throat / Diarrhea / Constipation

## FOR THE MEDICINAL HONEY

2 or 3 large lemons, sliced

1 (3- to 4-inch) piece of fresh ginger, sliced

1 (3- to 4-inch) piece of fresh turmeric, sliced

1 (22-ounce) jar raw organic honey

## FOR THE TEA

4 cups water

4 tablespoons dried chamomile flowers

SUBSTITUTION TIP: There are many herbs, in addition to chamomile, that are soothing and healing to the throat. Feel free to substitute with marshmallow root, slippery elm, licorice root, or fenugreek.

The honey in this magical tea tempers the spice of the ginger and turmeric, making it so sweet and drinkable that my children ask for it many mornings. This elixir is not only soothing but also provides nutrients that support the immune system, lower inflammation, and encourage healing of the delicate mucous membranes in your mouth and throat. Keep a jar of the medicinal honey at the ready so you can quickly make this tea anytime.

1. **Make the honey:** In a quart-size glass jar, alternate layers of the lemon, ginger, and turmeric slices until you get to the top of the jar. Pour the honey into the jar to cover the ingredients. If the honey is too thick to pour, place it in a pot of hot water until it loosens (do this only if the honey is in a glass jar).

2. Cover with a lid and refrigerate for at least 12 hours. (Can be refrigerated up to 1 month.)

3. **Make the tea:** Bring the water to a boil in a teapot or small saucepan. Turn off the heat, add the chamomile flowers, and cover. Steep for about 15 minutes.

4. Strain the liquid into 2 mugs. Add 2 tablespoons of medicinal honey to each mug, stir, and serve.

PER SERVING: Calories: 64; Total fat: 0g; Sodium: 1mg; Carbohydrates: 17g; Fiber: 0g; Protein: 0g

# Green Tea Detox

SERVES: 2 | PREP TIME: 5 Minutes | COOK TIME: 5 Minutes

SYMPTOMS: Nausea / Fatigue / Taste Changes / Unintentional Weight Loss / Diarrhea / Constipation

4 cups water
2 organic green tea bags
Juice of 1 lemon
2 teaspoons organic raw
    coconut oil

VARIATION TIP: You can use more or less coconut oil or lemon depending on your preference. You can also omit the coconut oil and just serve green tea and lemon juice. Alternatively, if you're experiencing mouth sores, omit the lemon and just serve green tea and coconut oil.

One of our most powerful cancer-healing foods, green tea supports detoxification, as well as being a rich source of anti-inflammatory and anticancer nutrients. Japanese varieties of green tea have the highest amounts of EGCG, a potent anticancer catechin. The lemon adds vitamin C and other immune-boosting antioxidants, while the coconut oil provides healthy fat and anti-microbial, digestive, and detox-supporting benefits. The coconut oil easily melts into the tea and is a great way to add more calories when you're looking to support weight gain.

1. Bring the water to a boil in a teapot or small saucepan.

2. Divide the boiling water between 2 mugs and add 1 tea bag to each mug. Steep for at least 5 minutes and up to 10 minutes to extract the most EGCG possible from the tea. Remove the tea bags and stir in the lemon juice and coconut oil. Serve immediately.

PER SERVING: Calories: 44; Total fat: 5g; Sodium: 0mg; Carbohydrates: 2g; Fiber: 0g; Protein: 0g

# Turmeric Milk

| SERVES: 2 | PREP TIME: 5 Minutes | COOK TIME: 10 Minutes |
|---|---|---|

SYMPTOMS: Nausea / Trouble Swallowing / Taste Changes /
Unintentional Weight Loss / Diarrhea / Constipation

2 cups unsweetened almond
milk or coconut milk
1 teaspoon ground turmeric
1 teaspoon ground cinnamon
½ teaspoon
ground cardamom
¼ teaspoon ground ginger
1 tablespoon honey or maple
syrup (optional)

The spices in this recipe imbue the milk with irresistible flavor, while adding healing, anti-inflammatory, anticancer, and immune-supporting nutrients. Turmeric milk also supports good digestion and can ease an upset stomach. If you're looking to add more calories, use canned full-fat coconut milk and add 1 tablespoon of coconut oil when heating.

In a small saucepan, combine the milk, turmeric, cinnamon, cardamom, and ginger over medium heat. Whisk together and bring to a low boil. Reduce the heat to low and simmer for 10 minutes. Strain into 2 mugs. Add the honey, if using, and serve.

SUBSTITUTION TIPS: If desired, use dairy milk instead of the plant-based milk here. Another option is to combine the ingredients in a blender, substituting a 1-inch piece of peeled fresh turmeric and a ½-inch piece of peeled fresh ginger for the ground spices. Blend until smooth and store in a glass bottle or jar in the refrigerator for up to 4 days. Enjoy cold or warm.

PER SERVING: Calories: 70; Total fat: 3g; Sodium: 150mg; Carbohydrates: 11g; Fiber: 1g; Protein: 1g

# Carrot, Beet, and Turmeric Juice

| MAKES: **3 to 4 Cups** | PREP TIME: **15 Minutes** | |

**SYMPTOMS:** Nausea / Fatigue / Anemia / Taste Changes / Diarrhea / Constipation

6 large carrots
2 medium green apples (such as Granny Smith), quartered
1 medium beet, halved
1 (1-inch) piece of fresh turmeric

The carrots and beets in this juice drink are powerful cancer-healing foods providing vitamins, minerals, antioxidants, and phyto-nutrients that support digestion, assist in detoxification, and lower inflammation. This recipe works best with a juicer. If you don't have one, use a high-speed blender or food processor and then strain the liquid through cheesecloth or a nut milk bag. Remember to wash your ingredients well. You do not need to peel them, but you can peel the beet if the taste is too earthy for you.

1. Run the carrots, apples, beets, and turmeric through a juicer, one at a time. If the pulp is still wet, you can re-juice by running the pulp back through the juicer.

2. Serve immediately for optimal nutrient and enzyme levels, or store in an airtight glass jar in the refrigerator for up to 24 hours.

SUBSTITUTION TIPS: Try using oranges (peeled) instead of the apples or fresh ginger instead of or in addition to the turmeric.

PER SERVING (1 CUP): Calories: 84; Total fat: 0g; Sodium: 100mg; Carbohydrates: 25g; Fiber: 1g; Protein: 2g

# Zesty Green Juice

| MAKES: **4 Cups** | PREP TIME: **15 Minutes** | |
|---|---|---|

SYMPTOMS: Fatigue / Taste Changes / Diarrhea / Constipation

1 large cucumber

6 fresh kale leaves

2 celery stalks

2 medium green apples (such as Granny Smith), quartered

½ lemon or 1 whole lime

1 (1-inch) piece of fresh ginger

If you're just getting started with juicing, consider making this easy green drink. All the ingredients support digestion, detoxification, and the immune system. This recipe works best with a juicer, but if you don't have a juicer, use a high-speed blender or food processor, then squeeze the liquid through cheesecloth or a nut milk bag. The pulp will be trapped in the cloth and you'll be left with clear juice. Wash your ingredients well. You do not need to peel any of them. If it's not too tart for you, including the lemon peel will provide important anticancer phytonutrients and essential oils.

1. Run the cucumber, kale, celery, apples, lemon half, and ginger through a juicer, one at a time. If the pulp is still wet, you can re-juice by running the pulp back through the juicer.

2. Serve immediately for optimal nutrient and enzyme levels or store in an airtight glass jar in the refrigerator for up to 24 hours.

SUBSTITUTION TIP: You can substitute any leafy green you have on hand for the kale, such as spinach, chard, bok choy, collards, or cabbage.

PER SERVING (1 CUP): Calories: 50; Total fat: 0g; Sodium: 22mg; Carbohydrates: 16g; Fiber: 0g; Protein: 3g

# Stomach-Soothing Juice

MAKES: **3 to 4 Cups** | PREP TIME: **15 Minutes**

SYMPTOMS: Nausea / Fatigue / Diarrhea / Constipation

½ bulb fennel

¼ cup fresh mint leaves and stems, tightly packed

1 large cucumber

2 celery stalks

2 medium green apples (such as Granny Smith), quartered

1 (1-inch) piece of fresh ginger

The fennel, mint, and ginger here are a perfect combination for digestive support. These ingredients help soothe an upset stomach; ease nausea, gas, or bloating; and support better digestion. This recipe works best with a juicer, but if you don't have a juicer, you can still make this in a high-speed blender or food processor, then squeeze the liquid through cheesecloth or a nut milk bag. The pulp will be trapped in the cloth and you'll be left with clear juice. Wash your ingredients well. You do not need to peel any of them.

1. Run the fennel, mint, cucumber, celery, apples, and ginger through a juicer, one at a time. If the pulp is still wet, you can re-juice by running the pulp back through the juicer.

2. Serve immediately for optimal nutrient and enzyme levels or store in an airtight glass jar in the refrigerator for up to 24 hours.

VARIATION TIP: Parsley, dandelion leaves, and cilantro are also herbs that help soothe the stomach and reduce gas or bloating. You can substitute these for the fennel and/or mint for a different take on this juice recipe.

PER SERVING (1 CUP): Calories: 40; Total fat: 0g; Sodium: 21mg; Carbohydrates: 13g; Fiber: 0g; Protein: 1g

# Anticancer Rainbow Smoothie

**30**

**V**

| SERVES: **2** | PREP TIME: **10 Minutes** | |
|---|---|---|

**SYMPTOMS:** Fatigue / Trouble Swallowing / Anemia / Unintentional Weight Loss / Constipation

2 cups fresh spinach or
   baby kale

½ cup fresh strawberries
   or raspberries

½ cup fresh blueberries
   or blackberries

1 small banana, peeled

1 small orange, peeled

1 (1-inch) piece of fresh
   ginger, peeled, or ½ teaspoon ground ginger

1 (1-inch) piece of fresh
   turmeric, peeled, or ½ teaspoon ground turmeric

½ teaspoon ground cinnamon

2 tablespoons raw
   almond butter

2 tablespoons chia seeds

2 cups water

A smoothie is the perfect quick, easy-to-digest meal that's full of fiber, protein, vitamins, and minerals. I have a general smoothie template I like to follow to keep it balanced: 2 cups veggies + 2 cups fruit + 2 tablespoons protein + 2 tablespoons healthy fat + 2 cups liquid. This recipe offers immune-boosting, anti-inflammatory, anticancer fruits and veggies from every color of the rainbow, in addition to healing spices.

1. In a high-speed blender or a food processor, blend the spinach, strawberries, blueberries, banana, orange, ginger, turmeric, cinnamon, almond butter, chia seeds, and water until smooth and creamy, 1 to 2 minutes.

2. Serve immediately or store in an airtight glass jar in the refrigerator for up to 2 days or in the freezer for up to 3 months.

PREP AHEAD TIP: You can store the mixture in pint-size mason jars in the freezer for several days. Take out your smoothie the night before and let it thaw in the refrigerator. When you're ready to drink, simply give it a good shake.

PER SERVING: Calories: 284; Total fat: 14g; Sodium: 12mg; Carbohydrates: 38g; Fiber: 13g; Protein: 8g

Drinks and Tonics   153

# Balanced Green Smoothie

| SERVES: 2 | PREP: 10 Minutes | |
|---|---|---|

SYMPTOMS: Fatigue / Trouble Swallowing / Anemia / Taste Changes / Unintentional Weight Loss / Constipation

2 cups fresh spinach or
    baby kale
1 small banana, peeled
½ cup chopped fresh or
    canned pineapple
½ cup chopped fresh or
    frozen mango
1 scoop organic hemp
    protein powder
½ avocado, pitted and peeled
2 cups water

This beginner-friendly green smoothie is perfectly balanced and sweet. It provides a great dose of fiber, protein, healthy fat, antioxidants, and anticancer nutrients. The smoothie supports a healthy immune system, and the consistency makes it easy to digest.

1. In a blender or a food processor, combine the spinach, banana, pineapple, mango, protein powder, avocado, and water until smooth and creamy, 1 to 2 minutes.

2. Serve immediately or store in an airtight glass jar in the refrigerator for up to 2 days or in the freezer for up to 3 months.

VARIATION TIP: To add more calories or protein to this smoothie, simply increase the amount of protein powder and avocado.

PER SERVING: Calories: 276; Total fat: 9g; Sodium: 191mg; Carbohydrates: 37g; Fiber: 9g; Protein: 16g

# Nourishing High-Calorie Smoothie

SERVES: **2** | PREP: **10 Minutes**

SYMPTOMS: Fatigue / Trouble Swallowing / Anemia / Unintentional Weight Loss / Constipation

1 ripe pear, cored and quartered

3 Medjool dates, pitted and chopped

2 cups frozen cauliflower florets

2 tablespoons raw cashew butter or other nut butter

¼ cup raw walnut pieces

2 tablespoons cacao nibs or powder

2 tablespoons organic raw coconut oil

2 cups unsweetened almond milk or coconut milk

Instead of reaching for a milkshake or a canned protein drink, consider making this sweet and healthy smoothie. The frozen cauliflower makes it extra creamy while also providing anticancer, detox-supporting, hormone-balancing benefits. The walnuts, nut butter, and coconut oil offer healthy anti-inflammatory fat calories, and the pear and dates give extra sweetness plus fiber.

1. In a high-speed blender or food processor, combine the pear, dates, cauliflower, cashew butter, walnuts, cacao nibs, coconut oil, and almond milk until smooth and creamy, 1 to 2 minutes.

2. Serve immediately or store in an airtight glass jar in the refrigerator for up to 2 days or in the freezer for up to 3 months.

FLAVOR BOOST TIP: I always love adding spices to my smoothies for both flavor and a health boost. Try adding fresh ginger (1 inch, peeled) or ½ teaspoon of ground cinnamon. Don't be afraid to experiment with different herbs and spices in your smoothies.

PER SERVING: Calories: 560; Total fat: 35g; Sodium: 187mg; Carbohydrates: 62g; Fiber: 11g; Protein: 11g

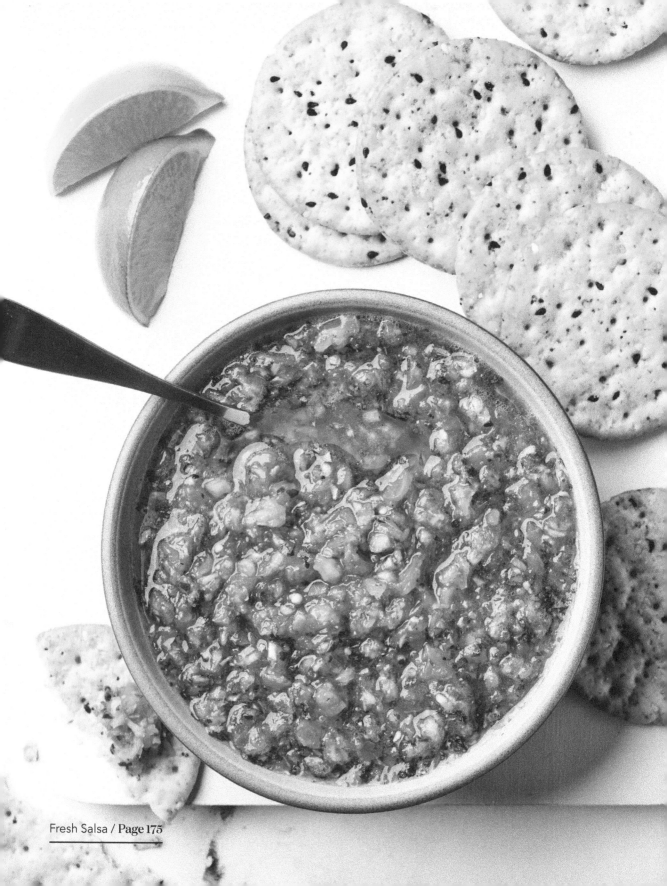

Fresh Salsa / **Page 175**

# CHAPTER 8

# Broths, Dressings, and Sauces

# Mineral-Rich Vegetable Broth

**MAKES:** 4 Quarts | **PREP:** 10 Minutes | **COOK:** 6 Hours (Stovetop) **or** 45 Minutes (Pressure Cooker)

**SYMPTOMS:** Nausea / Fatigue / Trouble Swallowing / Sore Mouth or Throat / Diarrhea / Constipation

2 medium onions
½ head garlic
4 large carrots,
   roughly chopped
2 large parsnips,
   roughly chopped
6 celery stalks with leaves,
   roughly chopped
1 large piece of kombu
1 (2-inch) piece of fresh ginger
1 (2-inch) piece of
   fresh turmeric
1 tablespoon
   black peppercorns
5 quarts filtered water

Even without added bones, this broth provides a multitude of vitamins, minerals, and nutrients. Kombu, a type of dried seaweed that's a rich source of antioxidants and even omega-3 fatty acids, can be found in Japanese markets, health food stores, and the international section of many grocery stores. But if you can't find it, don't worry; the broth will still be rich in minerals even without it. No peeling is involved here, but make sure all your vegetables are cleaned. You can make this broth on the stovetop or in an electric pressure cooker; there are instructions for both options.

### STOVETOP INSTRUCTIONS

1. Put the onions, garlic, carrots, parsnips, celery, kombu, ginger, turmeric, and peppercorns in a Dutch oven or large, deep pot and cover with the water, stopping 1 inch or so from the top.

2. Bring to a boil over high heat, then reduce the heat to low, cover, and simmer until the broth is fragrant and flavorful, 4 to 6 hours.

3. Cool to room temperature, then pour through a fine-mesh strainer into quart-size mason jars, allowing 2 to 3 inches expansion space at the top (if freezing). Discard the vegetables.

4. Store in the refrigerator for up to 1 week or in the freezer for up to 6 months.

## ELECTRIC PRESSURE COOKER INSTRUCTIONS

1. Place the onions, garlic, carrots, parsnips, celery, kombu, ginger, turmeric, and peppercorns in the cooker and cover with the water.

2. Secure the lid and cook on high pressure for 20 minutes. Allow the pressure to release naturally, then remove the lid.

3. Let the broth cool to room temperature, then pour through a fine-mesh strainer into quart-size mason jars, allowing 2 to 3 inches expansion space at the top (if freezing). Discard the vegetables.

4. Store in the refrigerator for up to 1 week or in the freezer for up to 6 months.

PREP AHEAD TIP: If desired, you can save your vegetable kitchen scraps (carrot peels and tops, celery trimmings, onion peels, parsnip peels, turnip trimmings, extra fresh herbs) in an airtight container in the freezer until you're ready to make broth.

PER SERVING (1 CUP): Calories: 10; Total fat: 0g; Sodium: 20mg; Carbohydrates: 3g; Fiber: 0g; Protein: 0g

# Mineral-Rich Bone Broth

| MAKES: **4 Quarts** | PREP: **10 Minutes** | COOK: | **5 Hours** (Stovetop) **or** **2 Hours** (Pressure Cooker) |

SYMPTOMS: Nausea / Fatigue / Trouble Swallowing / Sore Mouth or Throat / Diarrhea / Constipation

1 chicken carcass

¼ cup apple cider vinegar

1 medium onion

½ head garlic

2 large carrots,
  roughly chopped

1 large parsnip,
  roughly chopped

4 celery stalks with leaves,
  roughly chopped

1 large piece of kombu

1 (2-inch) piece of fresh ginger

1 (2-inch) piece of
  fresh turmeric

1 tablespoon
  black peppercorns

5 quarts filtered water

Bone broth is my absolute favorite recommendation for cancer patients. This hydrating liquid is full of easy-to-assimilate minerals, amino acids, and other nutrients that support the immune system and improve the health of your gut. It's my go-to recipe when clients don't feel like eating but need to stay hydrated, and it's the perfect fluid to consume when fasting. Make sure all the vegetables are cleaned before adding them to the pot. You can make this broth on the stovetop or in an electric pressure cooker; there are instructions for both options.

STOVETOP INSTRUCTIONS

1.  In a Dutch oven or large, deep pot, place the chicken carcass and pour the vinegar over it. Add the onion, garlic, carrots, parsnip, celery, kombu, ginger, turmeric, and peppercorns and cover with the water, stopping 1 inch or so from the top.

2.  Bring to a boil over high heat, then reduce the heat to low, cover, and simmer until the broth is rich and fragrant and the bones easily fall apart, at least 5 hours and up to 24 hours.

3. Let the broth cool to room temperature. Pour through a fine-mesh strainer into quart-size mason jars, leaving 2 to 3 inches at the top to allow for expansion (if freezing). Discard the vegetables and bones.

4. Store in the refrigerator for up to 1 week or in the freezer for up to 6 months.

## ELECTRIC PRESSURE COOKER INSTRUCTIONS

1. Place the chicken carcass in the cooker and pour the vinegar over it. Add the onion, garlic, carrots, parsnip, celery, kombu, ginger, turmeric, and peppercorns and cover with the water.

2. Secure the lid and cook on high pressure for 90 minutes. Allow the pressure to release naturally, then remove the lid.

3. Let the broth cool to room temperature, then pour through a fine-mesh strainer into quart-size mason jars, leaving 2 to 3 inches at the top to allow for expansion (if freezing). Discard the vegetables and bones.

4. Store in the refrigerator for up to 1 week or in the freezer for up to 6 months.

PREP AHEAD TIP: I like to keep 1 quart of broth in the refrigerator, ready to use, and store the others in the freezer. You can also consider freezing some of your broth in ice cube trays to more easily use small portions; each cube provides about 2 tablespoons of broth.

PER SERVING (1 CUP): Calories: 16; Total fat: 1g; Sodium: 40mg; Carbohydrates: 1g; Fiber: 0g; Protein: 1g

# Basic Chicken Bone Broth

MAKES: **4 Quarts** | PREP: **5 Minutes** | COOK: **5 Hours** (Stovetop) **or** **2 Hours** (Pressure Cooker)

SYMPTOMS: Nausea / Fatigue / Trouble Swallowing / Sore Mouth or Throat / Diarrhea / Constipation

1 chicken carcass
¼ cup apple cider vinegar
5 quarts filtered water

Basic bone broths are very easy to make, and they're great for gut health, as well as offering inflammation and immune support. You can use this simple chicken broth in any recipe that calls for broth, or you can warm it up and simply sip "as is" for another source of hydration. Bone broths don't require the addition of vegetables to the pot, but you can include them if you want to. The broth can be made on the stovetop or in an electric pressure cooker; there are instructions for both options.

## STOVETOP INSTRUCTIONS

1. In a Dutch oven or large, deep pot, place the chicken carcass and pour the vinegar over it. Cover with the water, stopping 1 inch or so from the top.

2. Bring to a boil over high heat, then reduce the heat to low, cover, and simmer for at least 5 hours and up to 24 hours.

3. Let the broth cool to room temperature, then pour through a fine-mesh strainer into quart-size mason jars, leaving 2 to 3 inches at the top of the jar to allow for expansion (if freezing). Discard the bones.

4. Store in the refrigerator for up to 1 week or in the freezer for up to 6 months.

ELECTRIC PRESSURE COOKER INSTRUCTIONS

1. Place the chicken carcass in the cooker, pour the vinegar over it, and cover with the water.

2. Secure the lid and cook on high pressure for 90 minutes. Allow the pressure to release naturally, then remove the lid.

3. Let the broth cool to room temperature, then pour through a fine-mesh strainer into quart-size mason jars, leaving 2 to 3 inches at the top of the jar to allow for expansion (if freezing). Discard the bones.

4. Store in the refrigerator for up to 1 week or in the freezer for up to 6 months.

PER SERVING (1 CUP): Calories: 13; Total fat: 1g; Sodium: 40mg; Carbohydrates: 0g; Fiber: 0g; Protein: 1g

# Basic Beef Bone Broth

| MAKES: **4 Quarts** | PREP: **5 Minutes** | COOK: | **24½ Hours** (Stovetop) |
|---|---|---|---|
| | | | **or 2½ Hours** (Pressure Cooker) |

**SYMPTOMS:** Fatigue / Trouble Swallowing / Sore Mouth or Throat / Diarrhea / Constipation

4 pounds beef soup bones (such as marrow bones and joint bones)

¼ cup apple cider vinegar

5 quarts filtered water

Beef broth has long been used as a healing beverage. It's a rich source of collagen, amino acids, glucosamine, chondroitin, and more. It's soothing and nourishing for the gut and a great way to boost hydration. Whenever possible, use bones from organic pasture-raised meat. You can make this broth on the stovetop or in an electric pressure cooker; there are instructions for both options. Just make sure you don't skip the first step of roasting the bones, as this builds the flavor of the broth.

### STOVETOP INSTRUCTIONS

1. Preheat the oven to 400°F. Lightly grease a baking sheet or roasting pan.

2. Place the bones in the pan and roast until well browned, 30 to 40 minutes.

3. In a Dutch oven or large, deep pot, place the bones and pour the vinegar over them. Cover with the water, stopping 1 inch or so from the top.

4. Bring to a boil over high heat, then reduce the heat to low, cover, and simmer for 24 hours. (If the broth ends up being too strong in flavor for you, the next time you make it, cook it for less time. Aim for a minimum of 12 hours.)

5. Let the broth cool to room temperature, then pour through a fine-mesh strainer into quart-size mason jars, leaving 2 to 3 inches at the top of the jar to allow for expansion (if freezing). Discard the bones.

6. Store in the refrigerator for up to 1 week or in the freezer for up to 6 months. When ready to use, be sure to spoon off the hard layer of fat on top. You can save the fat for cooking or discard it.

## ELECTRIC PRESSURE COOKER INSTRUCTIONS

1. Preheat the oven to 400°F. Lightly grease a baking sheet or roasting pan.

2. Place the bones in the pan and roast until well browned, 30 to 40 minutes.

3. Place the roasted bones in the cooker. Pour the vinegar over the bones and add the water.

4. Secure the lid and cook on high pressure for 90 minutes. Allow the pressure to release naturally, then remove the lid.

5. Let the broth cool to room temperature, then pour through a fine-mesh strainer into quart-size mason glass jars, leaving 2 to 3 inches at the top to allow for expansion (if freezing). Discard the bones.

6. Store in the refrigerator for up to 1 week or in the freezer for up to 6 months.

PER SERVING (1 CUP): Calories: 16; Total fat: 1g; Sodium: 38mg; Carbohydrates: 0g; Fiber: 0g; Protein: 2g

# Basic Fish Broth

| MAKES: **4 Quarts** | PREP TIME: **5 Minutes** | COOK TIME: **20 Minutes** |
|---|---|---|

SYMPTOMS: Nausea / Fatigue / Trouble Swallowing / Sore Mouth or Throat / Diarrhea / Constipation

4 pounds fish heads, back-bones, and trimmings
¼ cup apple cider vinegar
5 quarts filtered water

VARIATION TIP: You can also make this broth with the shells from shrimp, crab, lobster, and other shellfish. First roast the shells (about 2 pounds worth) in a single layer on a baking sheet in a 400°F oven for about 20 minutes, until they are browned and crispy. Then transfer the shells to the pot along with the vinegar and water. Slowly bring the broth to a simmer and then cook for about 45 minutes.

Fish bones cook very quickly and yield a nutrient-rich broth that can be enjoyed on its own or as the basis for light soups, like the Miso Soup with Tofu and Greens (page 102). This broth is best made with less oily fish, such as cod, trout, or snapper. You may, however, need to purchase a whole fish, unless your market sells fish heads for soup. To collect enough bones to make this broth, store the bones from cooked whole fish in an airtight container in the freezer for up to 6 months.

1. In a Dutch oven or large, deep pot, place the fish trimmings and pour the vinegar over them. Cover with the water, stopping 1 inch or so from the top.

2. Slowly bring the broth to a simmer over medium heat and continue to simmer for 20 to 30 minutes, until the broth is fragrant but not too strong. Let it cool to room temperature, then pour through a fine-mesh strainer into quart-size mason jars, leaving 2 to 3 inches at the top of the jar to allow for expansion (if freezing). Discard the bones.

3. Store in the refrigerator for up to 1 week or in the freezer for up to 6 months.

PER SERVING (1 CUP): Calories: 11; Total fat: 1g; Sodium: 37mg; Carbohydrates: 0g; Fiber: 0g; Protein: 1g

# Balsamic Vinaigrette

MAKES: **3 Cups** | PREP TIME: **10 Minutes**

SYMPTOMS: Taste Changes / Unintentional Weight Loss

1 cup balsamic vinegar
1 tablespoon Dijon mustard
2 garlic cloves, minced
   or pressed
¼ teaspoon sea salt
2 cups extra-virgin olive oil

If you're not already making your own salad dressing, it's time to start. Most bottled dressings have added sugar, salt, or other preservatives, but when you make your own you have control over the quality of ingredients. In addition to adding flavor, dressings offer healthy calories plus another avenue to bring in immune-boosting, anti-inflammatory, and anticancer nutrients. This dressing was inspired by my mother-in-law's classic French vinaigrette. We always have a bottle of it ready to go in the refrigerator.

In a glass jar with a tight-fitting lid, combine the vinegar, mustard, garlic, salt, and olive oil. Screw on the lid, then shake until thoroughly combined. Use immediately or store in the refrigerator for up to 2 weeks.

PER SERVING (2 TABLESPOONS): Calories: 169; Total fat: 18g; Sodium: 29mg; Carbohydrates: 2g; Fiber: 0g; Protein: 0g

# Lemon-Garlic Dressing

**MAKES: 1½ Cups** | **PREP TIME: 10 Minutes**

**SYMPTOMS:** Nausea / Taste Changes / Unintentional Weight Loss

Juice of 2 large lemons
2 garlic cloves, minced
  or pressed
¼ teaspoon sea salt
⅛ teaspoon freshly ground
  black pepper
1 cup extra-virgin olive oil

This dressing adds a delicious kick to salads along with a potent hit of vitamin C, among other nutrients. Both the citrus and the garlic support detoxification, digestion, and the immune system.

In a glass jar with a tight-fitting lid, combine the lemon juice, garlic, salt, pepper, and olive oil. Screw on the lid and shake until thoroughly combined. Use immediately or store in the refrigerator for up to 2 weeks.

**VARIATION TIP:** This recipe is equally delicious made with the juice of 4 small limes.

PER SERVING (2 TABLESPOONS): Calories: 162; Total fat: 18g; Sodium: 39mg; Carbohydrates: 1g; Fiber: 0g; Protein: 0g

# Honey Mustard Dressing

MAKES: **1 Cup**  |  PREP TIME: **10 Minutes**

SYMPTOMS: Nausea / Taste Changes / Unintentional Weight Loss

½ cup extra-virgin olive oil

¼ cup prepared
yellow mustard

4 tablespoons raw honey

3 tablespoons freshly
squeezed lemon juice

1 garlic clove, minced
or pressed

¼ teaspoon sea salt

⅛ teaspoon freshly ground
black pepper

The honey in this dressing provides antioxidants and antimicrobial benefits, while the lemon and garlic offer immune-boosting nutrients in addition to supporting digestion and detoxification. This dressing is the perfect choice when you're craving a sweeter option for your greens than the typical vinaigrette.

In a glass jar with a tight-fitting lid, combine the olive oil, mustard, honey, lemon juice, garlic, salt, and pepper. Screw on the lid and shake until thoroughly combined. Use immediately or store in the refrigerator for up to 2 weeks.

PER SERVING (2 TABLESPOONS): Calories: 158; Total fat: 14g; Sodium: 145mg; Carbohydrates: 10g; Fiber: 0g; Protein: 0g

# Creamy Turmeric Dressing

**MAKES: 1 Cup** | **PREP TIME: 10 Minutes**

**VG**

**SYMPTOMS:** Taste Changes / Sore Mouth or Throat / Unintentional Weight Loss

½ cup raw tahini
½ cup extra-virgin olive oil
2 tablespoons lemon juice
2 teaspoons raw honey
1 tablespoon ground turmeric
½ teaspoon sea salt
¼ teaspoon freshly ground
   black pepper

Bottled creamy dressings are often loaded with unhealthy calories—yet another reason to make your own. In addition to providing healthy fat, tahini is a good source of protein, iron, calcium, magnesium, and B vitamins. And as you likely know by now, turmeric is one of our most potent cancer-protective spices that also lowers inflammation, boosts the immune system, and supports both digestion and detoxification.

Whisk the tahini, olive oil, lemon juice, honey, turmeric, salt, and pepper in a small bowl until thoroughly combined. Store in an airtight glass jar in the refrigerator for up to 1 week.

PER SERVING (2 TABLESPOONS): Calories: 218; Total fat: 21g; Sodium: 134mg; Carbohydrates: 6g; Fiber: 2g; Protein: 3g

# Avocado-Cilantro Dressing

5

30

VG

| MAKES: **1 Cup** | PREP TIME: **10 Minutes** | |

**SYMPTOMS:** Trouble Swallowing / Taste Changes / Sore Mouth or Throat / Unintentional Weight Loss

1 medium avocado, pitted and peeled

1 garlic clove, peeled

¼ cup roughly chopped fresh cilantro

¼ cup plain full-fat Greek yogurt

¼ cup extra-virgin olive oil

1 tablespoon freshly squeezed lime juice

¼ teaspoon sea salt

¼ teaspoon freshly ground black pepper

¼ cup filtered water, or as needed

It's easy to incorporate more fresh herbs into your diet when you've got this versatile avocado-cilantro dressing in the fridge. Cilantro is a rich source of antioxidants, as well as anti-inflammatory and anticancer phytonutrients, and it supports good digestion and detoxification. To keep this dressing vegan, you can substitute a plant-based alternative for the yogurt.

In a food processor or blender, combine the avocado, garlic, cilantro, yogurt, olive oil, lime juice, salt, and pepper. Process until smooth and creamy, stopping to scrape down the sides as needed. Thin the dressing to a thick but pourable consistency by slowly adding the water, as much as needed. Store in an airtight glass jar in the refrigerator for up to 1 week.

**SUBSTITUTION TIP:** Although I personally love cilantro, I know not everybody does. This recipe works equally well with basil, mint, or flat-leaf parsley.

PER SERVING (2 TABLESPOONS): Calories: 111; Total fat: 11g; Sodium: 63mg; Carbohydrates: 4g; Fiber: 2g; Protein: 1g

# Basil-Spinach Pesto

| MAKES: **3 Cups** | PREP TIME: **10 Minutes** | |
|---|---|---|

SYMPTOMS: Fatigue / Trouble Swallowing / Taste Changes / Unintentional Weight Loss / Constipation

2 cups fresh basil leaves, tightly packed

1 cup fresh spinach, tightly packed

2 garlic cloves, peeled

1 cup extra-virgin olive oil, or more as needed

¼ cup pine nuts

½ teaspoon sea salt

½ cup grated Parmesan cheese (optional)

Pesto is the perfect medium to add more leafy greens, healthy fats, antioxidants, and plenty of immune-boosting, anti-inflammatory, anticancer nutrients to your diet. This recipe shows you how to make a classic basil pesto with the addition of spinach, but this is only one of many pesto versions you can make. One of my favorite resources for creative and delicious herbal pesto recipes is *The Herbal Kitchen* by Kami McBride; she devotes a whole chapter just to pesto.

In a food processor or blender, combine the basil, spinach, garlic, olive oil, pine nuts, salt, and Parmesan, if using. Process until thick and creamy, about 2 minutes. You can add more olive oil if needed to thin the sauce. Store in an airtight glass jar in the refrigerator for up to 1 week or in the freezer for up to 6 months.

VARIATION TIP: There are many different herbs, nuts, and seeds you can use to make pesto. Don't be afraid to experiment. The basic template is 3 cups herbs + 2 garlic cloves + 1 cup olive oil + ¼ to ½ cup nuts or seeds + ½ teaspoon sea salt.

PER SERVING (¼ CUP): Calories: 180; Total fat: 20g; Sodium: 80mg; Carbohydrates: 1g; Fiber: 0g; Protein: 1g

# Moroccan Marinade

**MAKES:** ¼ Cup  |  **PREP TIME:** 5 Minutes

**SYMPTOMS:** Nausea / Taste Changes

2 teaspoons ground cumin

1½ teaspoons ground ginger

1 teaspoon sea salt

1 teaspoon ground turmeric

1 teaspoon ground paprika

½ teaspoon ground cinnamon

½ teaspoon freshly ground
black pepper

2 tablespoons extra-virgin
olive oil

4 garlic cloves, minced
or pressed

The spices in this blend are full of immune-boosting and anti-inflammatory phytonutrients, and they also provide protective antioxidants, which are especially important when grilling meat. Cooking animal foods at high temperatures creates carcinogenic compounds. This reaction starts to happen above 212°F and becomes extremely dangerous above 500°F. Using a marinade with herbs and spices has been shown to decrease the formation of these dangerous compounds. In addition, spices like ginger can help calm nausea, while also enhancing flavor, which can help with taste changes.

In a small bowl, mix the cumin, ginger, salt, turmeric, paprika, cinnamon, pepper, olive oil, and garlic until a paste forms.

**PREP TIP:** Thoroughly coat the meat of choice with the marinade and marinate in the refrigerator for at least 30 minutes before grilling, or 15 minutes before cooking on the stovetop. This recipe makes enough to marinate 6 chicken thighs.

PER SERVING (2 TEASPOONS): Calories: 50; Total fat: 5g; Sodium: 314mg; Carbohydrates: 2g; Fiber: 1g; Protein: 0g

# Herbal Citrus Marinade

**MAKES: 1 Cup**  |  **PREP TIME: 10 Minutes**

**SYMPTOMS:** Nausea / Taste Changes

Grated zest and juice of
   1 large lime
Grated zest and juice of
   1 large lemon
Juice of 1 large orange
4 garlic cloves, minced
   or pressed
1 tablespoon minced
   fresh flat-leaf parsley, or
   1 teaspoon dried
1 tablespoon minced
   fresh rosemary, or
   1 teaspoon dried
1 tablespoon minced fresh
   thyme, or 1 teaspoon dried
1 tablespoon minced fresh
   basil, or 1 teaspoon dried
1 tablespoon minced fresh
   sage, or 1 teaspoon dried

Cooking meat with natural antioxidants greatly decreases or even eliminates carcinogenic by-products that come from high heat cooking. According to some studies, all herbs and spices offer some protection, with certain herbs like rosemary and thyme having the greatest effect. This tasty marinade combines potent antioxidant herbs with fresh citrus. Citrus flavors can be helpful for calming nausea, while the combination of citrus, garlic, and herbs enhances flavor, which can ease taste changes.

In a medium bowl, mix the lime and lemon zest and juice, orange juice, garlic, parsley, rosemary, thyme, basil, and sage. To use, pour the marinade into a large plastic bag, add the meat of choice, and seal the bag. Marinate for at least 30 minutes in the refrigerator before cooking.

PER SERVING (2 TEASPOONS): Calories: 4; Total fat: 0g; Sodium: 0mg; Carbohydrates: 1g; Fiber: 0g; Protein: 0g

# Fresh Salsa

| MAKES: **3 to 4 Cups** | PREP TIME: **10 Minutes** |
|---|---|

**SYMPTOMS:** Taste Changes / Constipation

Although this healthy and flavorful Mexican staple is synonymous with tacos, you might also enjoy it as an accompaniment to fish, chicken, or eggs, or as a dip for tortilla chips or raw vegetables. A word of caution: use a plastic baggie or disposable gloves to handle the hot peppers and wash your hands thoroughly with soap and hot water afterward. Avoid touching your eyes for several hours. Set aside some of the seeds from the peppers. If the salsa isn't hot enough, you can add a few later on for more heat.

4 ripe medium tomatoes (about 1¼ pounds), roughly chopped

½ red onion, roughly chopped

1 garlic clove, roughly chopped

1 jalapeño pepper or 2 serrano peppers, seeded

and roughly chopped (reserve seeds)

Juice of 1 lime

⅓ to ½ cup chopped fresh cilantro

¼ teaspoon dried oregano, crumbled

¼ teaspoon ground cumin

¼ teaspoon sea salt

⅛ teaspoon freshly ground black pepper

¼ to ½ teaspoon ground red chile (optional)

Chips, raw vegetables, or whole-grain crackers

1. In a food processor, combine the tomatoes, onion, garlic, jalapeño, lime juice, cilantro, oregano, cumin, salt, pepper, and ground chile, if using. Pulse several times, just enough to dice the ingredients but not enough to puree. (If you don't have a food processor, you can finely dice by hand.)

2. Place in a serving bowl and adjust seasonings as desired. (If too hot, add more tomato or ½ teaspoon of sugar; if not hot enough, add a few reserved seeds from the peppers.) Let the salsa sit for 1 hour in the refrigerator for the flavors to meld.

3. Serve as a dip with chips, vegetables, or crackers. Store in an airtight container in the refrigerator for up to 1 week.

PER SERVING (¼ CUP): Calories: 12; Total fat: 0g; Sodium: 51mg; Carbohydrates: 3g; Fiber: 1g; Protein: 0g

# Healthy Homemade Mayonnaise

MAKES: **1 Cup** | PREP TIME: **5 Minutes** | //////////////////

SYMPTOMS: Trouble Swallowing / Sore Mouth or Throat / Unintentional Weight Loss

1 pasteurized large egg yolk

1 tablespoon apple
cider vinegar

1 tablespoon freshly squeezed
lemon juice

1 teaspoon Dijon
mustard (optional)

1 garlic clove, minced or
pressed (optional)

¾ cup avocado or extra-virgin
olive oil

Sea salt

SUBSTITUTION TIP: This
recipe can easily be made
vegan. Substitute 7 ounces of
organic silken or soft tofu for the
egg yolk and blend as directed.

Store-bought mayonnaise options generally contain inflammatory oil, added sugar, and preservatives. But this version provides healthy anti-inflammatory fat with no added sugar or artificial ingredients. Adding mayonnaise to your meals and snacks is an easy and tasty way to boost calories when you're trying to maintain your weight, and the mayo can also add some moistness to your foods, which will make eating easier if you're having trouble swallowing.

1. Have all your ingredients at room temperature. Place the egg yolk, vinegar, lemon juice, and mustard and garlic, if using, in a food processor or blender and blend until smooth. (Alternatively, place everything in a small bowl and blend with an immersion blender or hand mixer.)

2. With the blender running, slowly add the oil in a thin, steady stream. Stop blending once the mayonnaise is thick and creamy. (Refrain from re-blending, as this can cause the mayonnaise to break.)

3. Add salt to taste. Use immediately or store in an airtight glass jar in the refrigerator for up to 1 week.

PER SERVING (1 TABLESPOON): Calories: 95; Total fat: 10g; Sodium: 14mg; Carbohydrates: 0g; Fiber: 0g; Protein: 0g

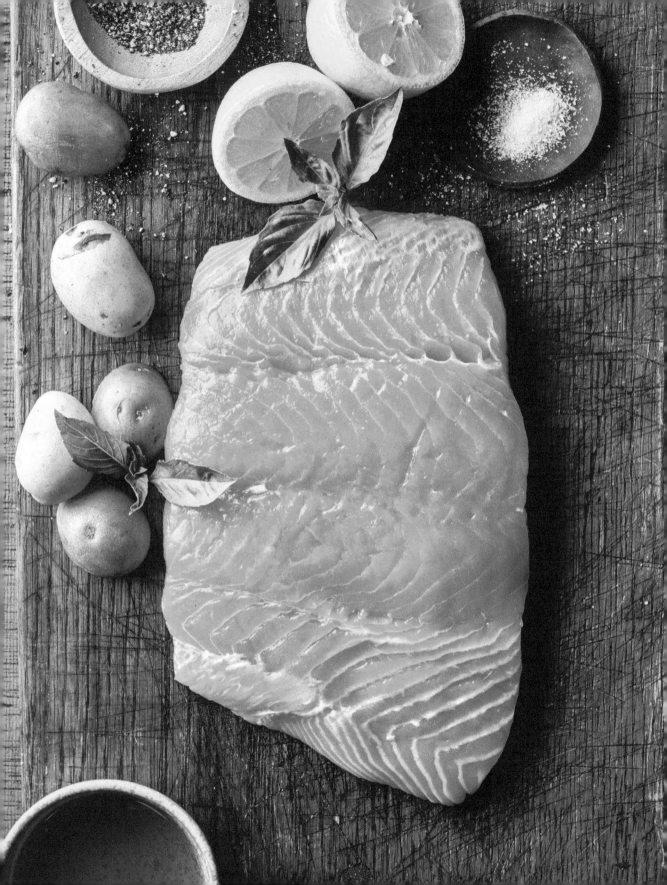

# MEASUREMENT CONVERSIONS

| Volume Equivalents | U.S. STANDARD | U.S. STANDARD (ounces) | METRIC (approximate) |
|---|---|---|---|
| **Liquid** | 2 tablespoons | 1 fl. oz. | 30 mL |
| | ¼ cup | 2 fl. oz. | 60 mL |
| | ½ cup | 4 fl. oz. | 120 mL |
| | 1 cup | 8 fl. oz. | 240 mL |
| | 1½ cups | 12 fl. oz. | 355 mL |
| | 2 cups or 1 pint | 16 fl. oz. | 475 mL |
| | 4 cups or 1 quart | 32 fl. oz. | 1 L |
| | 1 gallon | 128 fl. oz. | 4 L |
| **Dry** | ⅛ teaspoon | – | 0.5 mL |
| | ¼ teaspoon | – | 1 mL |
| | ½ teaspoon | – | 2 mL |
| | ¾ teaspoon | – | 4 mL |
| | 1 teaspoon | – | 5 mL |
| | 1 tablespoon | – | 15 mL |
| | ¼ cup | – | 59 mL |
| | ⅓ cup | – | 79 mL |
| | ½ cup | – | 118 mL |
| | ⅔ cup | – | 156 mL |
| | ¾ cup | – | 177 mL |
| | 1 cup | – | 235 mL |
| | 2 cups or 1 pint | – | 475 mL |
| | 3 cups | – | 700 mL |
| | 4 cups or 1 quart | – | 1 L |
| | ½ gallon | – | 2 L |
| | 1 gallon | – | 4 L |

## Oven Temperatures

| FAHRENHEIT | CELSIUS (approximate) |
|---|---|
| 250°F | 120°C |
| 300°F | 150°C |
| 325°F | 165°C |
| 350°F | 180°C |
| 375°F | 190°C |
| 400°F | 200°C |
| 425°F | 220°C |
| 450°F | 230°C |

## Weight Equivalents

| U.S. STANDARD | METRIC (approximate) |
|---|---|
| ½ ounce | 15 g |
| 1 ounce | 30 g |
| 2 ounces | 60 g |
| 4 ounces | 115 g |
| 8 ounces | 225 g |
| 12 ounces | 340 g |
| 16 ounces or 1 pound | 455 g |

# RESOURCES

There are many informative resources available to help guide your cancer-healing journey. In addition to my website, therusticdietitian.com, the following are some sources I find valuable and often share with my clients.

American Institute for Cancer Research website: aicr.org

*Anticancer: A New Way of Life*, by David Servan-Schreiber

*Anticancer Living: Transform Your Life and Health with the Mix of Six*, by Lorenzo Cohen and Alison Jefferies

*Foods to Fight Cancer: Essential Foods to Help Prevent Cancer*, by Richard Beliveau and Denis Gingras

*Radical Remission: Surviving Cancer Against All Odds*, by Kelly A Turner

UCSF Osher Center for Integrative Medicine: Cancer and Nutrition website: osher.ucsf.edu/patient-care/integrative-medicine-resources/cancer-and-nutrition

The World's Healthiest Foods website: whfoods.com

# INDEX

# ACKNOWLEDGMENTS

I first need to thank my husband, Marc, who took over all the house chores, grocery shopping, playdates, many meals, and much more so that I could have the space and time I needed to write this book. I also want to thank my daughters, Lola and Teah, for being so understanding and giving me uninterrupted time to write, as well as being willing to test many of the recipes in this book and sharing their "honest" feedback.

I want to thank my friends and family who shared their favorite recipes to help fuel my inspiration, specifically Rebecca Mullen, Izaskun Uriz, and Morgan Patton. I am also especially grateful to my clients and the Rustic Dietitian community who have used many of these recipes during their own healing journeys and shared their valuable feedback.

A huge thank you to Callisto Media for giving me the opportunity to write this book and to share these recipes with you. To my managing editor, Greg Morabito, for being so kind, supportive, and generous with his time throughout the entire process and to my development editor, Gabriella Gershenson, for so thoroughly reviewing and offering her expert guidance with all the recipes.

Finally, I will forever be grateful to my dad who showed me how to be brave, resilient, and optimistic throughout both of his bouts with cancer. It was because of his journey and all that I learned along the way that I am here today sharing this work with you.

# ABOUT THE AUTHOR

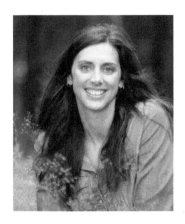

**Dionne Detraz, RDN,** is an Integrative Dietitian with over a decade of experience supporting people through their cancer journeys. She has worked in hospitals and at an integrative medicine clinic, and currently supports people through her online practice and website, therusticdietitian.com. She believes wholeheartedly in the power of food and integrative strategies to support healing, and has dedicated her life to helping others optimize their cancer recovery with these tools. Originally from California, Dionne lives with her husband and their two daughters in France.

CPSIA information can be obtained
at www.ICGtesting.com
Printed in the USA
JSHW052321250822
29603JS00002B/6